The Ultimate Fitness Handbook: Transform Your Life

Kevin D. Harper

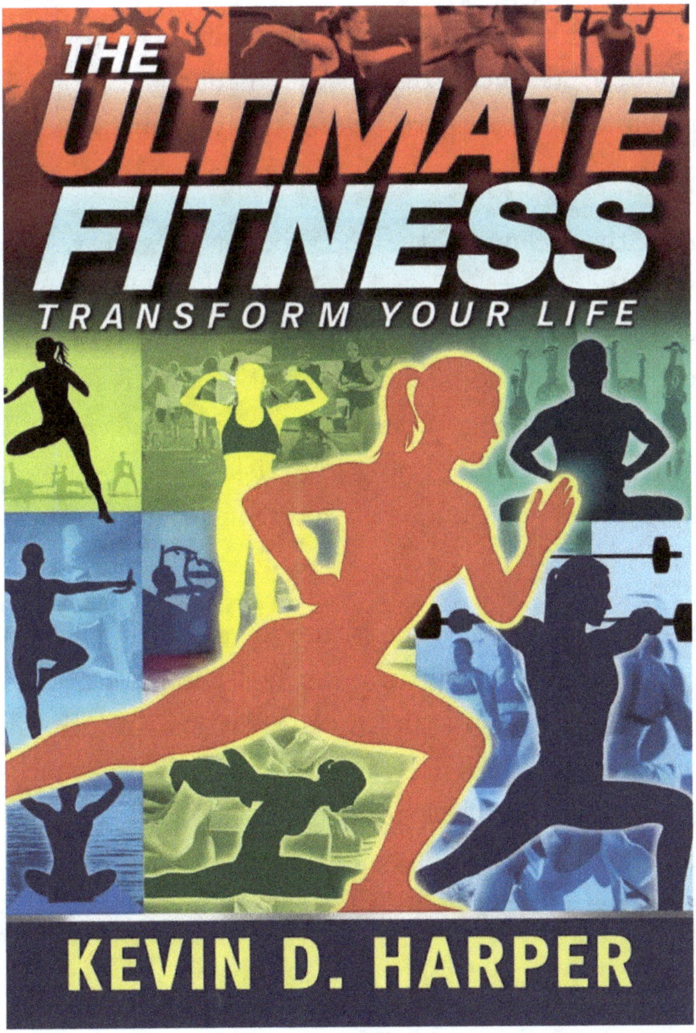

Copyright © by Kevin D. Harper

Introduction

Welcome to The Ultimate Fitness Handbook: Transform Your Life by Kevin D. Harper, your guide to achieving a healthier, stronger, and more confident version of yourself. Whether you're just starting your fitness journey or looking to take your results to the next level, this book will help you unlock your true potential. The fitness world can be overwhelming with endless information, trends, and conflicting advice. So, how do you cut through the noise and find what works? That's where The Ultimate Fitness Handbook comes in. It clarifies your fitness journey, providing proven strategies and techniques that work for everyone, regardless of age, fitness level, or experience.

This book is based on years of research, expert knowledge, and real-life experiences. It takes a holistic approach to fitness, focusing on exercise, nutrition, mindset, and recovery. Here's a quick look at what you'll discover:

- **Step-by-Step Exercise Plans:** Tailored routines for beginners to advanced athletes.

- **Nutrition for Peak Performance:** Simple, actionable advice on fueling your body.

- **Mindset Mastery:** Techniques for building mental toughness and staying motivated.

- **Recovery Strategies:** How to rest and recover to maximize your results.

Imagine transforming your body and life, feeling more assertive, energized, and confident in your skin. This book gives you the tools to make that vision a reality. Applying the strategies within these pages will give you the knowledge, discipline, and motivation needed to overcome obstacles and achieve long-lasting results.

It's time to stop making excuses and start making progress. Let The Ultimate Fitness Handbook be your companion on this journey toward a healthier, happier you. Begin reading now, and take your first step toward transformation. Your future self will thank you. Let's get started! Your ultimate fitness journey begins now.

Table of Contents

Chapter 1: Introduction to Fitness and Wellness

Fitness and wellness are foundational aspects of human health that influence every facet of life, from physical capabilities to mental clarity. This chapter introduces the concept of fitness, explores its significance in ensuring overall well-being, and delves into the intricate relationship between physical and psychological health. Additionally, it highlights the idea of holistic fitness, emphasizing the integration of various dimensions of health to achieve optimal living.

Defining Fitness and Its Importance for Overall Well-being

What Is Fitness?

Fitness refers to the ability of an individual to perform daily activities with vigor and alertness, without undue fatigue, and with sufficient energy to enjoy leisure-time pursuits and meet unforeseen emergencies. It encompasses multiple dimensions, including cardiovascular endurance, muscular strength, flexibility, and body composition.

1. **Physical Fitness:**
    - Physical fitness is often categorized into health-related and skill-related components.
    - Health-related fitness includes cardiovascular endurance, muscular strength, endurance, flexibility, and body composition. These elements contribute to the functional health necessary for everyday life.
    - Skill-related fitness focuses on agility, balance, coordination, power, reaction time, and speed, which are more specific to athletic performance.
2. **Mental Fitness:**
    - Mental fitness pertains to cognitive and emotional well-being. It involves maintaining a state of mental clarity, focus, and emotional stability.
    - It enables individuals to handle stress, make sound decisions, and maintain a positive outlook on life.

Why Is Fitness Important?

1. **Physical Benefits:**
    - Enhances cardiovascular and muscular health.
    - Reduces the risk of chronic illnesses such as heart disease, diabetes, and obesity.
    - Improves immune function, helping the body fend off diseases.
    - Increases longevity and the quality of life.
2. **Mental and Emotional Benefits:**
    - Regular physical activity stimulates the release of endorphins, chemicals in the brain that act as natural painkillers and mood elevators.
    - Reduces symptoms of anxiety, depression, and stress.

- Boosts self-esteem and self-confidence, fostering a positive self-image.

3. **Social Benefits**:
   - Encourages participation in group activities, fostering a sense of community and belonging.
   - Promotes better communication and social interactions.

4. **Cognitive Benefits**:
   - Enhances brain function, memory, and concentration.
   - Delays in cognitive decline associated with aging.

5. **Economic Benefits**:
   - Reduces healthcare costs by preventing lifestyle-related diseases.
   - Improves productivity at work by enhancing physical and mental energy.

The Relationship Between Physical and Mental Health

Physical and mental health are deeply intertwined, creating a feedback loop where each influences the other.

1. **Physical Activity as a Mental Health Booster**:
   - Exercise has been shown to improve mood and reduce symptoms of depression and anxiety. It achieves this by:
     - Increasing blood circulation to the brain impacts stress responses.
     - Promoting neurogenesis, the growth of new brain cells, particularly in areas associated with memory and emotion.

2. **The Impact of Mental Health on Physical Health**:
   - Chronic stress can lead to physical ailments such as high blood pressure, heart disease, and weakened immune function.
   - Mental health conditions like depression often result in sedentary behavior, poor eating habits, and disrupted sleep, all of which negatively affect physical health.

3. **The Role of the Mind-Body Connection**:
   - The mind-body connection emphasizes how mental states can influence physical health. For instance, mindfulness practices have been linked to reduced inflammation and improved cardiovascular health.
   - Techniques such as yoga, tai chi, and meditation integrate physical activity with mental focus, enhancing physical and psychological well-being.

4. **Neurochemical Mechanisms**:
   - Physical activity influences brain chemicals, such as serotonin, dopamine, and endorphins, which regulate mood and motivation.
   - Similarly, mental health interventions can alter hormonal responses, like cortisol reduction, benefiting physical health.

Introducing the Concept of Holistic Fitness

Holistic fitness goes beyond traditional definitions of physical fitness, incorporating mental, emotional, social, and spiritual dimensions. It recognizes that well-being is multi-faceted and interconnected.

1. **Components of Holistic Fitness:**
   - **Physical Health:**
     - Engaging in regular exercise tailored to individual needs.
     - Ensuring proper nutrition to fuel the body and promote recovery.
   - **Mental Health:**
     - Practicing mindfulness and stress management techniques.
     - Engaging in activities that challenge the mind, such as puzzles, reading, or creative hobbies.
   - **Emotional Health:**
     - Developing emotional intelligence and resilience.
     - Building healthy coping mechanisms to manage life's challenges.
   - **Social Health:**
     - Cultivating supportive relationships.
     - Participating in community activities to foster a sense of belonging.
   - **Spiritual Health:**
     - Exploring personal values and purpose.
     - Engaging in practices like meditation, prayer, or connecting with nature.

2. **Benefits of Holistic Fitness:**
   - Promotes balance across various aspects of life.
   - Reduces the risk of burnout by addressing both physical and mental needs.
   - Enhances adaptability to life's challenges by fostering a well-rounded sense of resilience.

3. **Practical Applications of Holistic Fitness:**
   - Incorporating diverse types of exercise, such as aerobic activities, strength training, and flexibility exercises.
   - Maintaining a balanced diet rich in nutrients while acknowledging the role of hydration.

- Prioritizing mental health practices, including therapy, journaling, or meditation.
- Building meaningful relationships and participating in social networks that support growth and well-being.
- Creating a spiritual practice that aligns with personal beliefs through traditional religious frameworks or secular practices.

Modern Perspectives on Fitness and Wellness

1. **Technological Advances:**
   - Fitness tracking devices and apps provide real-time physical activity and health metrics feedback.
   - Virtual fitness programs and online communities have made holistic fitness more accessible.

2. **Cultural Shifts:**
   - There is growing recognition of the importance of mental health, with many organizations offering resources to support holistic well-being.
   - Wellness tourism and retreats focus on integrating fitness, nutrition, mental health, and spirituality.

3. **Challenges in Achieving Fitness and Wellness:**
   - Sedentary lifestyles and increased screen time contribute to physical and mental health issues.
   - Economic and social barriers prevent some populations from accessing fitness and wellness resources.

4. **The Role of Education:**
   - Educating individuals about the principles of fitness and wellness fosters lifelong healthy habits.
   - Schools and workplaces are increasingly incorporating wellness programs to promote holistic health.

Conclusion

The introduction to fitness and wellness underscores these aspects' critical role in achieving a fulfilling and healthy life. Understanding the definition of fitness and its impact on overall well-being sets the stage for exploring more complex interactions between physical and mental health. By embracing holistic fitness, individuals can ensure balance across the various dimensions of health, fostering resilience and adaptability in an ever-changing world.

Chapter 2: Setting Realistic Goals

Embarking on a journey toward fitness, personal development, or any significant lifestyle change requires a strong foundation of well-thought-out goals. This chapter focuses on setting realistic goals using the SMART framework, emphasizing the importance of tracking progress, adjusting goals as needed, and discovering personal motivation to maintain long-term commitment.

2.1 The Process of Setting SMART Goals

The SMART framework—Specific, Measurable, Achievable, Relevant, and Time-bound—provides a clear and structured goal-setting approach. Each component ensures that goals are actionable and attainable, fostering a sense of direction and purpose. Let's break down each element in detail:

1. **Specific**
2. Goals must be clear and precise, leaving no room for ambiguity. Vague goals such as "I want to lose weight" or "I want to be fit" lack direction. Instead, a specific goal might be, "I want to lose 10 pounds in three months by exercising three times a week and following a balanced diet."
   - **Why it's essential**: Specific goals provide focus, making it easier to devise actionable steps.
   - **Practical Tip**: Define what you want to achieve, why it matters, and how to accomplish it.
3. **Measurable**
4. To track progress effectively, goals should have quantifiable outcomes. This allows you to quantify your efforts and celebrate small milestones.
   - **Example**: Instead of saying, "I want to get stronger," aim for "I want to increase my bench press by 20 pounds within two months."
   - **Why it's essential**: Measurement creates accountability and gives you a clear sense of achievement.
   - **Practical Tip**: Use metrics like weight, reps, time, or frequency to measure your progress.
5. **Achievable**
6. While ambitious goals can be inspiring, unrealistic ones may lead to frustration and burnout. Goals should challenge you but remain within the realm of possibility.
   - **Example**: If you've never run before, setting a goal to run a marathon within two months is unrealistic. A more achievable goal might be completing a 5K within eight weeks.

- **Why it's essential**: Achievable goals build confidence and prevent discouragement.
- **Practical Tip**: Assess your current abilities and resources before setting your target.

7. **Relevant**
8. Your goals should align with your broader aspirations, values, and priorities. A goal that holds personal significance is more likely to motivate you.
   - **Example**: If your primary aim is improving cardiovascular health, focusing on endurance-based activities like running or cycling is more relevant than prioritizing weightlifting.
   - **Why it's essential**: Relevant goals ensure your efforts are meaningful and impactful.
   - **Practical Tip**: Reflect on why the goal matters and how it fits into your vision.

9. **Time-bound**
10. Goals need a deadline to create a sense of urgency and maintain momentum. An open-ended goal may lead to procrastination.
    - **Example**: "I will lose 5 pounds by the end of the month" is more effective than "I will lose weight eventually."
    - **Why it's essential**: Deadlines help prioritize actions and create a structured timeline.
    - **Practical Tip**: Break larger goals into smaller time-bound milestones for sustained progress.

2.2 The Importance of Tracking Progress and Adjusting Goals

Setting goals is only the beginning; monitoring progress and adjusting are equally critical for long-term success. Progress tracking allows you to evaluate what's working, identify areas for improvement, and stay motivated.

1. **Tracking Progress**
2. Tracking provides tangible evidence of improvement and helps you stay accountable.
   - **Methods:**
     - Maintain a journal to record workouts, meals, and achievements.
     - Use fitness apps or wearable devices to monitor activity levels, calorie intake, and other metrics.
     - Take regular photos or measurements to track changes visually.
   - **Why it's essential**: Seeing evidence of progress reinforces positive behaviors and fosters a sense of accomplishment.

3. **Adjusting Goals**

4. Life is dynamic, and unforeseen challenges can arise. Flexibility in adjusting goals ensures that setbacks don't derail your journey.
    - **Examples**:
        - If an injury prevents you from running, focus on low-impact exercises like swimming or yoga.
        - If weight loss slows, re-evaluate your diet and exercise routine to identify areas for improvement.
    - **Why it's essential**: Adjustments keep you on track, allowing you to adapt to changing circumstances without losing sight of your ultimate goal.
5. **Celebrating Milestones**
6. Recognizing and celebrating small achievements along the way boosts motivation and confidence.
    - **Example**: Treat yourself to new workout gear or a healthy meal after reaching a milestone.
    - **Why it's essential**: Acknowledging progress prevents burnout and maintains enthusiasm.

2.3 Finding Personal Motivation for Fitness

Motivation is the driving force behind any goal. While external factors like social pressure or rewards can kickstart your journey, lasting success comes from intrinsic motivation—your internal reasons for pursuing a goal.

1. **Understanding Your "Why"**
2. Reflect on why fitness matters to you personally.
    - **Examples**:
        - Improving health to avoid chronic illnesses.
        - Gaining energy to keep up with your children.
        - Boosting self-confidence and mental well-being.
    - **Why it's important**: A solid personal "why" serves as a reminder during challenging times.
3. **Setting Emotionally Resonant Goals**
4. Emotionally resonant goals are more potent than superficial ones.
    - **Example**: Instead of focusing solely on aesthetics, emphasize benefits like feeling strong, reducing stress, or increasing stamina.
    - **Why it's essential**: Meaningful goals create more profound commitment and satisfaction.
5. **Visualizing Success**
6. Visualization techniques can enhance motivation by helping you imagine the rewards of achieving your goal.
    - **Practice**: Spend a few minutes each day visualizing yourself succeeding, whether crossing a finish line or fitting into a favorite outfit.

- **Why it's essential**: Positive imagery reinforces belief in your ability to succeed.

7. **Building a Support System**
8. Surrounding yourself with supportive individuals can amplify motivation.
   - **Examples**:
     - Join fitness groups or classes to connect with like-minded individuals.
     - Share your goals with friends or family for encouragement.
   - **Why it's important**: A strong support network provides accountability and emotional reinforcement.
9. **Focusing on the Journey, Not Just the Destination**
10. Enjoying the process is crucial for long-term commitment.
    - **Examples**:
      - Experiment with different workouts to find activities you genuinely enjoy.
      - Appreciate non-scale victories like improved mood, energy, or sleep.
    - **Why it's important**: A positive mindset fosters sustainability and reduces the likelihood of burnout.

Conclusion

Setting realistic goals is the cornerstone of any successful endeavor. The SMART framework ensures that goals are well-defined and actionable while tracking progress and adjusting strategies keeps you on course. Ultimately, discovering and nurturing personal motivation transforms the journey into a fulfilling experience, ensuring lasting success and growth. By embracing these principles, readers can confidently embark on their fitness journey, knowing they have the tools to achieve their aspirations.

Chapter 3: Understanding Your Body

This chapter is a deep dive into understanding the human body as it relates to fitness. It is divided into three main sections: the basics of human anatomy, the influence of body types on fitness, and the significance of recognizing one's limits and potential. By the end of this chapter, readers will have a clearer understanding of how their unique physiology impacts their fitness journey and how they can use this knowledge to achieve better results.

Section 1: Basics of Human Anatomy Related to Fitness

Human anatomy forms the foundation of fitness. Understanding how the body is structured and functions can help you tailor workouts to achieve specific goals, prevent injuries, and maximize results. Below, we will explore the critical components of anatomy that are most relevant to fitness:

1.1 Muscular System

The muscular system is vital in movement, strength, and endurance. It consists of three main types of muscles:

- **Skeletal Muscles:** These are the muscles we train during workouts. They are responsible for voluntary movements, such as lifting weights or running. Skeletal muscles are further categorized into:
    - **Type I (Slow-Twitch) Fibers:** Designed for endurance, these fibers are predominant in long-distance running or cycling activities.
    - **Type II (Fast-Twitch) Fibers:** These fibers are responsible for explosive power and speed and dominate activities like sprinting and weightlifting.
- **Smooth Muscles:** Found in the walls of internal organs, these muscles work involuntarily to regulate digestion and blood flow.
- **Cardiac Muscle:** Exclusive to the heart, this muscle pumps blood throughout the body and is strengthened through cardiovascular exercises.

Understanding muscle anatomy allows individuals to effectively target specific muscle groups. Compound exercises like squats engage multiple muscle groups, while isolation exercises like bicep curls focus on a single muscle.

1.2 Skeletal System

The skeletal system provides structure, supports movement, and protects vital organs. Critical aspects of the skeletal system relevant to fitness include:

- **Joints:** There are three types of joints:
    - **Fixed Joints:** Found in the skull, these joints do not allow movement.
    - **Cartilaginous Joints:** Partially movable, such as those in the spine.
    - **Synovial Joints:** Fully movable joints like the knee, elbow, and shoulder. These are critical in fitness as they allow a range of motion.

- **Bones:** Weight-bearing exercises such as running or resistance training can increase bone density and reduce the risk of osteoporosis.
- **Alignment and Posture:** Proper posture and alignment prevent injury during exercise. For instance, maintaining a neutral spine during deadlifts reduces stress on the lower back.

1.3 Cardiovascular System

The cardiovascular system, comprising the heart and blood vessels, supplies oxygen and nutrients to muscles during exercise. It consists of:

- **Heart:** Regular exercise strengthens the heart, improves blood flow, and reduces the risk of cardiovascular diseases.
- **Blood Vessels:** Arteries, veins, and capillaries work together to deliver oxygen and remove waste products like carbon dioxide.

Cardiovascular health is critical for endurance-based activities. High-intensity interval training (HIIT) and steady-state cardio effectively improve cardiovascular fitness.

1.4 Respiratory System

The respiratory system works with the cardiovascular system to deliver oxygen to muscles and remove carbon dioxide. Key components include:

- **Lungs:** Efficient lung function ensures adequate oxygen supply during workouts.
- **Diaphragm:** Strengthening the diaphragm through breathing exercises can enhance performance and endurance.

1.5 Nervous System

The nervous system controls muscle activation and coordination. It includes:

- **Central Nervous System (CNS):** The brain and spinal cord coordinate movement and response to exercise.
- **Peripheral Nervous System (PNS):** Transmits signals between the CNS and muscles, enabling quick reactions.

Activities like plyometric training enhance neuromuscular coordination, leading to improved athletic performance.

1.6 Metabolic Systems

The body uses three central energy systems during exercise:

- **Phosphagen System:** Provides immediate energy for short, high-intensity efforts like sprinting.
- **Glycolytic System:** Supplies energy for moderate-intensity efforts lasting up to two minutes.
- **Oxidative System:** Powers low-intensity, long-duration activities by using fat as fuel.

Section 2: Overview of How Different Body Types Affect Exercise and Results

No two bodies are the same. Body type, or somatotype, significantly influences how an individual responds to exercise, their natural strengths, and the areas they may need to focus on. There are three primary body types, though most people fall somewhere on a spectrum:

2.1 Ectomorph

- **Characteristics:**
  - Lean and slim with a low body fat percentage.
  - Narrow shoulders and hips.
  - Difficulty gaining weight or muscle.
- **Fitness Considerations:**
  - Focus on strength training to build muscle mass.
  - Consume a calorie-dense diet with high protein and complex carbohydrates.
  - Limit excessive cardio, as it can hinder muscle gain.
- **Advantages:**
  - Naturally efficient at endurance-based activities like long-distance running.
  - Less prone to storing body fat.

2.2 Mesomorph

- **Characteristics:**
  - Naturally muscular and athletic build.
  - Broad shoulders, narrow waist, and a balanced body composition.
  - Gains muscle and strength quickly.
- **Fitness Considerations:**
  - Can excel in both strength and endurance activities.
  - A balanced diet with moderate macronutrient intake supports optimal performance.
  - Variety in training ensures balanced muscle development.
- **Advantages:**
  - Quick responders to exercise programs.
  - Versatile and capable of excelling in multiple sports or fitness routines.

2.3 Endomorph

- **Characteristics:**
  - Stocky build with a higher body fat percentage.
  - Wider hips and a tendency to gain weight quickly.
- **Fitness Considerations:**
  - Prioritize cardiovascular exercises to burn fat.
  - Include strength training to preserve lean muscle mass.
  - Focus on a controlled-calorie diet with low sugar and refined carbohydrates.
- **Advantages:**
  - Naturally strong and powerful, making them well-suited for sports requiring brute strength.

Section 3: Importance of Knowing One's Limits and Potential

Fitness is not just about pushing boundaries; it's about understanding and respecting your body. Recognizing personal limits and potential ensures safe and effective progress.

3.1 Avoiding Overtraining

Overtraining can lead to injuries, burnout, and diminished results. Signs include chronic fatigue, decreased performance, and persistent muscle soreness. Strategies to avoid overtraining:

- Incorporate rest days into your routine.
- Listen to your body and scale back intensity when needed.
- Use periodization techniques, alternating between high- and low-intensity phases.

3.2 Setting Realistic Goals

Fitness goals should be Specific, Measurable, Achievable, Relevant, and Time-bound (SMART). Unrealistic expectations can lead to frustration and decreased motivation.

3.3 Importance of Flexibility and Mobility

Flexibility and mobility exercises improve joint health, posture, and performance. Techniques include:

- Dynamic stretching before workouts to warm up muscles.
- Static stretching after workouts to enhance recovery.
- Yoga or Pilates for overall flexibility and mental relaxation.

3.4 Understanding Genetics and Potential

Genetics plays a role in fitness potential, including muscle fiber composition, metabolism, and body fat distribution. While genetics set a baseline, consistent effort, and tailored training can lead to significant improvements.

3.5 Psychological Aspect of Fitness

Mental health is as important as physical health. Strategies to maintain a positive mindset include:

- Celebrating small victories.
- Practicing mindfulness and stress management.
- Seeking support from friends, trainers, or fitness communities.

Conclusion

Understanding your body is the cornerstone of a compelling fitness journey. Knowledge of anatomy helps you train smarter, awareness of body types allows you to personalize your routine, and recognizing your limits ensures long-term success. By aligning your fitness approach with your unique physiology, you can unlock your full potential while staying safe and motivated.

Chapter 4: Cardio Basics

Cardiovascular exercises, or cardio for short, form the backbone of fitness routines to enhance heart health, improve stamina, and achieve overall well-being. This chapter delves into the definition, benefits, types of cardio workouts, and practical guidelines to help individuals incorporate cardio safely and effectively into their daily lives.

1. **Definition and Benefits of Cardiovascular Exercises**

Definition of Cardiovascular Exercises

Cardiovascular exercises are physical activities that increase the heart and respiratory rates for an extended period. The primary goal is to improve the function of the cardiovascular system, which comprises the heart, lungs, and blood vessels. Commonly referred to as aerobic exercises, they rely on the consistent use of oxygen to fuel muscle activity, making them distinct from anaerobic exercises like weightlifting.

Critical characteristics of cardio:

- **Sustained Movement**: Running, cycling, or swimming involve continuous motion.
- **Moderate to High Intensity**: The intensity can vary depending on fitness goals and individual capacity.
- **Oxygen Utilization**: Energy is generated primarily through oxygen-dependent processes.

Benefits of Cardiovascular Exercises

The advantages of cardio exercises extend beyond physical fitness, impacting mental health and overall longevity.

1. **Heart Health**
   - Regular cardio strengthens the heart muscle, improving its efficiency in pumping blood.
   - It reduces the risk of cardiovascular diseases like hypertension, coronary artery disease, and stroke.
2. **Improved Lung Capacity**
   - Aerobic activities enhance the lungs' ability to take in and utilize oxygen efficiently.
   - Over time, this leads to better stamina and endurance.
3. **Weight Management**
   - Cardio burns calories, helping in weight loss or maintenance.
   - It boosts metabolism, allowing the body to burn calories even at rest.
4. **Mental Health Benefits**
   - Exercise triggers the release of endorphins, often called "feel-good" hormones.
   - It reduces symptoms of anxiety, depression, and stress.

5. **Blood Sugar and Cholesterol Regulation**
   - Cardio helps regulate blood sugar levels by improving insulin sensitivity.
   - It can increase HDL (good cholesterol) while lowering LDL (bad cholesterol).
6. **Enhanced Immune Function**
   - Moderate cardio boosts the immune system by promoting the circulation of white blood cells.
7. **Better Sleep**
   - People engaging in regular cardio often report improved sleep quality and duration.
8. **Different Types of Cardio Workouts**

Cardiovascular exercises are categorized into low-impact, high-impact, and interval-based workouts. The choice depends on an individual's fitness level, goals, and preferences.

Low-Impact Cardio Workouts

Low-impact exercises are gentle on the joints, making them suitable for beginners, older adults, or those recovering from injuries.

1. **Walking**
   - It is one of the most straightforward and most accessible forms of cardio.
   - Brisk walking can help improve cardiovascular health and aid weight loss.
2. **Swimming**
   - Provides a full-body workout with minimal stress on joints.
   - Particularly beneficial for individuals with arthritis or mobility issues.
3. **Cycling**
   - Engages the lower body muscles while being gentle on the knees.
   - It can be done outdoors or on stationary bikes indoors.
4. **Elliptical Training**
   - Combines the benefits of walking and climbing with reduced impact on joints.
   - Famous in gym settings for its versatility.

High-Impact Cardio Workouts

High-impact exercises are more intense and often involve both feet leaving the ground at some point. These are ideal for individuals aiming for maximum calorie burn or athletic conditioning.

1. **Running or Jogging**
   - Increases heart rate significantly and engages multiple muscle groups.

- It can be adapted for beginners (slow jogging) or advanced athletes (sprints).

2. **Jumping Rope**
   - Provides an efficient calorie burn in a short time.
   - Enhances coordination, agility, and lower-body strength.
3. **Aerobics or Dance Workouts**
   - Combines rhythmic movements with music for a fun, engaging workout.
   - Examples include Zumba or step aerobics.
4. **Stair Climbing**
   - Intensifies cardio training by adding a resistance element.
   - Targets the glutes, hamstrings, and calves.

Interval-Based Cardio Workouts

Interval training alternates between high-intensity bursts and low-intensity recovery periods. Known for its efficiency, this method can yield significant fitness improvements in less time.

1. **High-Intensity Interval Training (HIIT)**
   - Involves short, intense bursts of exercise followed by brief recovery periods.
   - For example, sprinting for 30 seconds, then walking for 1 minute.
2. **Circuit Training**
   - Combines cardio and strength exercises in a series of stations.
   - Examples include jumping jacks, burpees, and push-ups performed consecutively.
3. **Tabata Training**
   - A specific form of HIIT involves 20 seconds of intense activity followed by 10 seconds of rest, repeated for four minutes.

Recreational Cardio Activities

Some people prefer incorporating cardio through recreational sports or outdoor adventures, such as:
- Playing soccer, basketball, or tennis.
- Hiking or trekking.
- Kayaking or rowing.

1. **Guide to Getting Started with Cardio, Including Safety Tips**

Getting Started with Cardio

For those new to cardio or returning after a break, it's essential to start slow and build up gradually to avoid injuries and ensure long-term adherence.

1. **Set Realistic Goals**
   - Define your goal: weight loss, endurance, or general health.
   - Break larger goals into smaller milestones for motivation.

2. **Choose Activities You Enjoy**
   - Experiment with various types of cardio to find what suits your preferences.
   - Enjoyable activities increase the likelihood of consistency.
3. **Start Small**
   - Begin with shorter durations, such as 10-15 minutes daily, and gradually increase the time and intensity.
4. **Warm-Up and Cool Down**
   - Start with 5-10 minutes of light activity to prepare the body.
   - Finish with stretches to reduce muscle soreness and improve flexibility.
5. **Track Progress**
   - Use fitness apps, pedometers, or heart rate monitors to keep track of your workouts.
   - Celebrate small achievements to stay motivated.

Safety Tips

Safety should be a priority to prevent injuries and ensure a positive experience.

1. **Consult a Healthcare Professional**
   - If you have pre-existing medical conditions or are new to exercise, seek medical advice before starting.
2. **Invest in Proper Gear**
   - Wear appropriate footwear to provide adequate support and minimize joint strain.
   - Dress in breathable, moisture-wicking fabrics.
3. **Stay Hydrated**
   - Drink water before, during, and after workouts to prevent dehydration.
4. **Listen to Your Body**
   - Stop immediately if you experience dizziness, chest pain, or extreme fatigue.
   - Avoid overtraining by incorporating rest days.
5. **Adapt to Your Environment**
   - Choose safe locations for outdoor activities, avoiding high-traffic areas.
   - Adjust intensity based on weather conditions.
6. **Gradual Progression**

- Avoid increasing intensity or duration too quickly to reduce the risk of injuries.

7. **Follow Proper Form**

    - Incorrect technique can lead to muscle strain or joint problems.
    - Seek guidance from fitness professionals if needed.

Tips for Sustained Motivation

Maintaining enthusiasm for cardio can be challenging. Here are strategies to stay on track:

- **Buddy System**: Exercise with friends or family for accountability.
- **Variety**: Alternate between different cardio workouts to prevent boredom.
- **Music or Podcasts**: Create playlists or listen to podcasts during sessions.
- **Set Rewards**: Treat yourself to small rewards after achieving milestones.

Conclusion

Cardiovascular exercises are a cornerstone of physical and mental health, offering numerous benefits ranging from heart health to stress reduction. With a diverse range of options catering to various fitness levels and preferences, there's a suitable cardio workout for everyone. By starting gradually, following safety guidelines, and staying consistent, individuals can enjoy the transformative effects of regular cardio, paving the way for a healthier, more vibrant life.

Chapter 5: Strength Training Fundamentals

Strength training, also known as resistance training, is an essential component of fitness that promotes health, functional ability, and athletic performance. This chapter delves into the benefits of strength training, outlines fundamental exercises for different muscle groups, and explains the role of resistance in various forms.

1. Benefits of Strength Training for All Ages

Strength training benefits individuals of all ages, from children to older adults. This section explores the advantages beyond physical appearance, including health, mental well-being, and injury prevention.

1.1 Physical Benefits

- **Improved Muscle Strength:** Strength training increases muscles' force-producing capacity, enhancing daily functioning and physical performance.
- **Bone Density:** Regular resistance exercises help maintain or improve bone mineral density, reducing the risk of osteoporosis, especially in older adults.
- **Joint Health:** Strength training stabilizes joints and reduces the risk of injuries by strengthening muscles, tendons, and ligaments.
- **Weight Management:** Strength training boosts metabolism by increasing muscle mass, which burns more calories at rest.

1.2 Mental and Emotional Benefits

- **Stress Reduction:** Resistance training releases endorphins, improving mood and reducing anxiety and depression.
- **Enhanced Cognitive Function:** Studies suggest a positive correlation between strength training and improved memory, focus, and executive function in older adults.
- **Self-Esteem:** Achieving physical goals through strength training boosts self-confidence and body image.

1.3 Benefits Across Age Groups

- **Children and Adolescents:**
  - Develops foundational strength and coordination.
  - It supports proper growth and posture during the developmental years.
  - Helps combat obesity by promoting an active lifestyle.
- **Adults:**
  - Enhances athletic performance and supports long-term health.
  - Improves functional fitness, enabling the performance of daily tasks with ease.
- **Seniors:**
  - Slows down muscle atrophy associated with aging (sarcopenia).
  - Improves balance and reduces the risk of falls, a leading cause of injury in older adults.

1. Essential Strength Exercises for Different Muscle Groups

Practical strength training involves targeting major muscle groups through compound and isolation exercises. Each section below covers critical muscle groups and examples of exercises that enhance strength and functionality.

2.1 Chest (Pectoral Muscles)

- **Push-Ups:** Bodyweight exercise that targets the chest, shoulders, and triceps.
- **Bench Press:** Using a barbell or dumbbell to lift weight while lying on a bench.
- **Chest Fly:** Dumbbell or machine-based exercise focusing on pectoral isolation.

2.2 Back (Latissimus Dorsi, Trapezius, Erector Spinae)

- **Pull-Ups/Chin-Ups:** Bodyweight exercise that strengthens the lats and biceps.
- **Bent-Over Rows:** Targets the lats, rhomboids, and lower back using dumbbells or a barbell.
- **Deadlifts:** Compound lift that engages the lower back, glutes, hamstrings, and core.

2.3 Legs (Quadriceps, Hamstrings, Calves, Glutes)

- **Squats:** A foundational movement targeting the quads, glutes, hamstrings, and core.
- **Lunges:** Builds balance, coordination, and strength in the legs and hips.
- **Calf Raises:** Isolates the calf muscles for improved strength and endurance.

2.4 Shoulders (Deltoids)

- **Overhead Press:** A barbell or dumbbell exercise focusing on shoulder and triceps strength.
- **Lateral Raises:** Isolation exercise targeting the middle deltoids.
- **Face Pulls:** Strengthens the rear deltoids and improves posture.

2.5 Arms (Biceps, Triceps, Forearms)

- **Bicep Curls:** Isolation movement using dumbbells, cables, or resistance bands.
- **Triceps Dips:** Bodyweight exercise that strengthens the triceps.
- **Hammer Curls:** Targets both the biceps and forearms.

2.6 Core (Abdominals, Obliques, Lower Back)

- **Planks:** Static hold that strengthens the core and stabilizes muscles.
- **Russian Twists:** Rotational movement engaging the obliques.
- **Dead Bug:** Dynamic core exercise for stabilization and spinal health.

1. **Understanding Resistance (Weights, Bands, Bodyweight)**

Resistance is the critical strength training component, providing the necessary stimulus for muscle adaptation and growth. This section explores different types of resistance and their applications.

3.1 Free Weights

Free weights, including dumbbells, barbells, and kettlebells, are versatile tools for resistance training. They allow for a wide range of motion and engage stabilizing muscles.

- **Advantages:**
  - Encourages natural movement patterns.

* Builds overall stability and coordination.
        * Suitable for both beginners and advanced lifters.
    * **Applications:** Ideal for compound movements like squats, deadlifts, and bench presses.

3.2 Resistance Bands

Resistance bands are elastic bands that provide variable resistance throughout an exercise's range of motion. They are lightweight, portable, and cost-effective.

* **Advantages:**
        * Safer for beginners and rehabilitation exercises.
        * Allows for progressive overload by using bands of varying resistance levels.
        * Reduces joint strain due to low-impact nature.
    * **Applications:** Great for mobility drills, light resistance workouts, and accessory exercises.

3.3 Bodyweight Training

Bodyweight exercises use the individual's weight as resistance. This approach requires minimal equipment and is accessible to everyone.

* **Advantages:**
        * Promotes functional fitness by mimicking real-world movements.
        * Suitable for individuals of all fitness levels.
        * Improves relative strength (strength-to-bodyweight ratio).
    * **Applications:** Ideal for beginners and can be progressed through modifications (e.g., weighted vests, elevated platforms).

3.4 Machines

Strength training machines guide movements along a fixed path, reducing the risk of improper form.

* **Advantages:**
        * Excellent for beginners learning basic strength exercises.
        * Targets specific muscle groups for isolation.
        * Reduces the risk of injury by controlling the range of motion.
    * **Applications:** Effective for focused hypertrophy and rehabilitation exercises.

1. **Principles of Progressive Overload and Recovery**

Strength training is grounded in progressive overload, which states that muscles must be gradually challenged beyond their usual limits to grow and adapt.

4.1 Implementing Progressive Overload

* **Increase Resistance:** Gradually add more weight or resistance to exercises.
* **Increase Repetitions or Sets:** Perform more repetitions or add extra sets to a workout.
* **Modify Tempo:** Slow down or speed up movements to increase time under tension.
* **Vary Exercises:** Introduce new exercises to target muscles from different angles.

4.2 Importance of Recovery

Recovery is crucial for muscle repair, adaptation, and growth. Overtraining can lead to fatigue, injury, and diminished performance.

- **Rest Days:** Incorporate at least one or two rest days per week.
- **Nutrition:** Consume adequate protein, carbohydrates, and healthy fats to support muscle repair.
- **Sleep:** Aim for 7–9 hours of quality sleep to optimize recovery.
- **Active Recovery:** Encourage low-intensity activities like walking or yoga to promote blood flow.

1. **Common Misconceptions About Strength Training**

Strength training is often surrounded by myths that deter individuals from incorporating it into their fitness routines.

5.1 "Strength Training is Only for Athletes"

Fact: Strength training benefits everyone, regardless of athletic ability, by improving health, functionality, and longevity.

5.2 "Lifting Weights Makes Women Bulky"

Fact: Women typically have lower levels of testosterone than men, making it unlikely that they will develop bulky muscles. Instead, strength training promotes a lean and toned physique.

5.3 "Strength Training is Unsafe for Kids"

Fact: With proper supervision and age-appropriate exercises, strength training is safe and beneficial for children.

5.4 "Older Adults Should Avoid Strength Training"

Fact: Strength training is one of the most effective ways to counteract age-related muscle loss and maintain independence.

1. **Conclusion**

Strength training is a versatile and essential form of exercise that promotes physical, mental, and functional well-being. By understanding its benefits, practicing foundational exercises, and appropriately using resistance, individuals of all ages can enhance their quality of life. Adopting strength training as a lifelong practice builds a resilient body and fosters a healthier mind and spirit.

Chapter 6: Flexibility and Balance

Flexibility and balance are foundational components of physical fitness and critical to maintaining overall health and well-being. This chapter delves into the significance of these attributes, introduces practical exercises like yoga and Pilates, and outlines techniques for improving range of motion and balance.

Importance of Maintaining Flexibility and Balance

Flexibility refers to the ability of muscles and joints to move through their full range of motion. On the other hand, balance is the ability to maintain the body's center of gravity over its base of support, whether stationary or in motion. These two components are interconnected and essential for daily activities and athletic performance.

1. **Health Benefits of Flexibility**

Flexibility enhances mobility, prevents injuries, and alleviates muscle stiffness. Key benefits include:

- **Improved Posture:** Tight muscles can cause imbalances that lead to poor posture. Stretching helps maintain proper alignment.
- **Enhanced Athletic Performance:** A more excellent range of motion enables efficient movement during physical activities.
- **Reduced Risk of Injury:** Flexible muscles are less prone to strain, and a good range of motion can prevent joint-related injuries.
- **Alleviation of Pain:** Stretching can reduce muscle tension and chronic pain, especially in areas like the lower back, shoulders, and neck.

1. **Health Benefits of Balance**

Good balance is vital for preventing falls and maintaining coordination. It becomes increasingly essential with age:

- **Fall Prevention:** For older adults, balance training reduces the risk of falls, a leading cause of injury.
- **Core Strength Improvement:** Balance exercises strengthen core muscles, which support stability and posture.
- **Enhanced Coordination:** Improved balance translates to better body control during activities.

1. **Everyday Applications**

Flexibility and balance contribute to efficiency in everyday activities. Tasks such as bending to pick up objects, climbing stairs, or even walking require a blend of these capabilities. With sufficient flexibility, simple movements can become relaxed and comfortable.

Introduction to Exercises Like Yoga and Pilates

Yoga and Pilates are among the most effective exercise regimens for developing flexibility and balance. Both practices focus on controlled movements, mindfulness, and core stability, offering numerous physical and mental benefits.

1. **Yoga**

Yoga is an ancient practice that integrates physical postures (asanas), breathing techniques (pranayama), and meditation. It emphasizes mind, body, and spirit union while promoting flexibility and balance.

- **Flexibility Enhancement:** Yoga stretches and elongates muscles, improving overall flexibility. Poses such as the Downward Dog and Pigeon Pose are particularly effective for targeting tight areas like the hamstrings and hips.
- **Balance Improvement:** Many yoga poses challenge balance by requiring focus and coordination. Poses like the Tree Pose and Warrior III engage core muscles and improve proprioception.
- **Stress Reduction:** Yoga encourages relaxation, reduces muscle tension, improves body awareness, and indirectly enhances balance and flexibility.
- **Accessibility:** Yoga is adaptable to all fitness levels, making it suitable for beginners and advanced practitioners.

1. **Pilates**

Pilates, developed by Joseph Pilates in the early 20th century, is a low-impact exercise method emphasizing core strength, flexibility, and overall body awareness.

- **Core Focus:** Pilates strengthens deep core muscles essential for stability and balance.
- **Flexibility Improvement:** Pilates exercises, such as the Spine Stretch Forward and Saw, increase the range of motion in the spine and limbs.
- **Body Alignment:** Pilates encourages proper alignment, helping reduce muscular imbalances and improve posture.
- **Controlled Movements:** Unlike fast-paced workouts, Pilates prioritizes precision, ensuring each movement contributes to balance and flexibility.

Techniques for Improving Range of Motion and Balance

Incorporating specific techniques into a fitness routine can significantly enhance flexibility and balance. The following strategies offer a systematic approach to improvement:

1. **Dynamic Stretching**

Dynamic stretching involves active movements that take joints and muscles through their full range of motion. It's ideal as a warm-up before exercise.

- **Examples:** Arm circles, leg swings, and walking lunges.
- **Benefits:** Prepares the body for activity, increases blood flow to muscles, and enhances mobility.

1. **Static Stretching**

Static stretching involves holding a stretch for 20-30 seconds to lengthen muscles and improve flexibility. It's most effective after a workout.

- **Examples:** Hamstring stretch, quad stretch, and seated forward bend.
- **Benefits:** Improves flexibility over time and reduces muscle soreness.

1. **Proprioceptive Neuromuscular Facilitation (PNF)**

PNF is an advanced stretching technique involving alternating contraction and relaxation of muscles.

- **How It Works:** A muscle is stretched to its limit, then contracted against resistance, followed by further stretching.

- **Benefits:** Increases flexibility more effectively than static stretching alone.

1. **Balance-Specific Exercises**

Balance exercises challenge stability and improve coordination. They often engage the core and lower body muscles.

- **Examples:**
    - **Single-Leg Stands:** Stand on one leg for 30 seconds, gradually increasing the duration.
    - **Heel-to-Toe Walks:** Walk in a straight line, placing one foot directly in front of the other.
    - **BOSU Ball Exercises:** Perform squats or lunges on a BOSU ball to challenge stability.
- **Benefits:** Enhances coordination, strengthens stabilizing muscles, and reduces fall risk.

1. **Strength Training**

Strengthening muscles, particularly in the core and lower body, supports balance and stability.

- **Focus Areas:** Exercises like planks, squats, and lunges target muscles crucial for balance.
- **Benefits:** Increased muscle strength provides a stable foundation for movement.

1. **Mind-Body Practices**

Activities combining physical movement with mental focus, such as tai chi, enhance balance and flexibility.

- **Tai Chi:** A Chinese martial art characterized by slow, deliberate movements. It improves coordination, balance, and mental clarity.
- **Benefits:** Builds body awareness, enhances joint mobility, and reduces stress.

1. **Using Props**

Props like resistance bands, foam rollers, and stability balls can aid flexibility and balance training.

- **Resistance Bands:** Assist in deeper stretches and improve joint mobility.
- **Foam Rollers:** Help release tight muscles through self-myofascial release.
- **Stability Balls:** Add an element of instability to exercises, engaging core muscles.

Tips for Successful Training

To maximize results, consider the following guidelines:

1. **Consistency:** Regular practice is essential for sustained improvement in flexibility and balance.
2. **Gradual Progression:** Avoid pushing too hard too soon. Allow the body to adapt to new movements gradually.
3. **Warm-Up:** Always warm up before stretching to prevent injury and maximize muscle pliability.
4. **Mindfulness:** Attention to alignment, breathing, and body sensations during exercises.

5. **Variety:** Incorporate a mix of techniques, including yoga, Pilates, and strength training, to target different aspects of flexibility and balance.

Long-Term Benefits of Flexibility and Balance Training

Consistently working on flexibility and balance offers long-term advantages, including:

- **Enhanced Quality of Life:** Improved mobility and reduced risk of falls lead to greater independence and confidence in daily life.

- **Delayed Aging:** Flexibility and balance training can counteract age-related declines in mobility and coordination.

- **Better Athletic Performance:** Athletes benefit from increased range of motion, coordination, and body control.

- **Stress Reduction:** Mind-body practices contribute to mental well-being, complementing physical health.

Conclusion

Flexibility and balance are integral to a healthy and active lifestyle. Incorporating exercises like yoga and Pilates, along with targeted techniques for improving range of motion and stability, can yield significant physical and mental benefits. Whether for athletic performance, fall prevention, or daily functionality, prioritizing these components of fitness fosters resilience and well-being at every stage of life. By embracing a consistent and mindful approach, individuals can unlock their full potential and enjoy a more balanced and flexible existence.

Chapter 7: Creating a Personalized Workout Plan

Creating a personalized workout plan is one of the most effective ways to achieve fitness goals, whether building muscle, losing weight, improving endurance, or simply maintaining overall health. A personalized plan is tailored to your unique needs, lifestyle, and goals, ensuring maximum benefit from your workouts while minimizing the risk of injury or burnout. This chapter breaks down the process into three main sections: designing an effective plan, incorporating variety and gradual progression, and maintaining consistency.

1. **Steps to Designing an Effective Workout Plan According to Individual Needs**

Designing a workout plan that fits your personal needs requires a structured approach. Here's how you can create a compelling and sustainable workout regimen:

Step 1: Define Your Goals

- **Understand your priorities:** Identify your primary fitness goal. Common goals include weight loss, muscle gain, increasing strength, enhancing flexibility, or improving cardiovascular health.
- **Set SMART goals:** Goals should be Specific, Measurable, Achievable, Relevant, and Time-bound. For example, "I want to lose 10 pounds in three months by exercising five times weekly."

Step 2: Assess Your Current Fitness Level

- **Physical assessment:** Measure your current abilities, such as cardiovascular endurance, strength, flexibility, and body composition.
- **Lifestyle evaluation:** Consider your daily activity level, work schedule, and physical limitations or health conditions.

Step 3: Choose Appropriate Exercises

- **Cardiovascular activities:** For heart health and calorie burning, include running, cycling, swimming, or brisk walking.
- **Strength training:** Incorporate exercises that target major muscle groups, such as squats, deadlifts, push-ups, and bench presses.
- **Flexibility and mobility:** Add stretching routines or practices like yoga to improve your range of motion.
- **Functional movements:** Use compound exercises that mimic real-life actions to enhance functionality and prevent injuries.

Step 4: Structure Your Workouts

- **Frequency:** Decide how often you'll exercise per week. Beginners might start with 3–4 days, while more experienced individuals could work out 5–6 days a week.

- **Intensity:** Use the Rate of Perceived Exertion (RPE) scale or track your heart rate to ensure you work at the right intensity.
- **Time:** Allocate 30–60 minutes per session, depending on your schedule and goals.
- **Type:** Mix different types of exercise to ensure balanced development.

Step 5: Plan Recovery

- **Rest days:** Schedule at least one or two weekly rest days to allow your body to repair and recover.
- **Active recovery:** On recovery days, engage in low-intensity activities like walking or light stretching to promote blood flow and reduce soreness.

Step 6: Monitor and Adjust

- **Track progress:** Keep a journal or use fitness apps to log your workouts, track improvements, and identify areas needing adjustment.
- **Adapt as needed:** Regularly evaluate your plan and make modifications to ensure continued progress and alignment with your goals.

1. **Importance of Variety and Gradual Progression in Exercises**

Sticking to the same workout routine can lead to boredom, stagnation, and even performance plateaus. Variety and progression are vital to maintaining enthusiasm and achieving long-term results.

Why Variety Matters

- **Prevents boredom:** Changing up your exercises keeps workouts exciting and motivating.
- **Targets different muscles:** Introducing new exercises ensures that all muscle groups are engaged and prevents imbalances.
- **Reduces risk of injury:** Repeating the same motions can lead to overuse injuries. Variety distributes the workload across different joints and muscles.
- **Improves overall fitness:** Mixing aerobic, strength, and flexibility exercises create a well-rounded fitness profile.

How to Incorporate Variety

- **Change exercises:** Swap out movements regularly, such as switching from push-ups to bench presses for chest work.
- **Adjust equipment:** To keep things fresh, use different tools, such as free weights, resistance bands, or body weights.
- **Experiment with formats:** Try circuit training, high-intensity interval training (HIIT), or traditional steady-state cardio.
- **Alter environments:** Move from the gym to outdoor spaces or try virtual workout classes.

Importance of Gradual Progression Progression ensures continuous improvement while minimizing the risk of overtraining or injury. With progression, the body adapts to the workload, and improvements continue.

Principles of Progression

- **Progressive overload:** Gradually increase your workouts' intensity, volume, or duration. For instance, add weight to your lifts or extend your running distance by small increments.
- **Skill progression:** Start with simpler movements and progress to more complex exercises as your coordination improves.
- **Recovery balance:** Incorporate proper rest and avoid pushing too hard too quickly to allow time for adaptation.

Example of Gradual Progression

- Week 1: Perform 3 sets of 10 push-ups.
- Week 3: Increase to 4 sets of 12 push-ups.
- Week 5: Progress to decline push-ups or add resistance bands.

1. **Tips for Staying Consistent with a Workout Plan**

Consistency is often the most challenging aspect of any fitness journey. To make fitness a sustainable part of your lifestyle, you need strategies to overcome barriers and stay motivated.

Develop a Routine

- **Set a schedule:** Work out at the same time every day to create a habit. Morning workouts prevent distractions later in the day.
- **Prepare in advance:** Lay out your workout clothes and equipment the night before to eliminate excuses.

Stay Accountable

- **Track progress:** Use a fitness app or journal to monitor your achievements and stay motivated by seeing how far you've come.
- **Find a workout buddy:** Exercising with a friend or joining a fitness community can provide mutual encouragement and accountability.

Stay Flexible

- **Adapt to life's demands:** If you miss a session, don't dwell on it. Adjust your schedule and keep moving forward.
- **Have a backup plan:** Have short, home-based workouts ready for days when time is limited.

Focus on Enjoyment

- **Do what you love:** Choose activities that you genuinely enjoy, whether it's dance, hiking, or team sports.
- **Reward yourself:** Celebrate milestones with non-food rewards like new workout gear or a spa day.

Manage Mindset

- **Set realistic expectations:** Understand that progress is gradual and avoid comparing yourself to others.

- **Reframe setbacks:** View missed workouts or indulgences as learning opportunities rather than failures.

Use Motivation Techniques

- **Visualize success:** Picture yourself achieving your fitness goals and the benefits it will bring.

- **Create a vision board:** Include images and quotes that inspire you to stay on track.

- **Mix up the motivation:** Listen to energetic playlists, watch inspiring fitness videos, or read success stories.

Make It Convenient

- **Eliminate obstacles:** Join a gym near your home or workplace or invest in home equipment to save time.

- **Incorporate mini-sessions:** Break your workout into shorter segments throughout the day if you're busy.

Conclusion

Creating a personalized workout plan is an empowering step towards achieving your fitness aspirations. By following the outlined steps, incorporating variety and progression, and maintaining consistency, you'll see physical benefits and experience improved mental health and confidence. Remember, your journey is unique; your plan should reflect your needs and preferences. Adjust as necessary, enjoy the process, and celebrate every milestone.

Chapter 8: Building Healthy Habits

Creating a sustainable and healthy lifestyle is not just about making decisions; it's about forming habits that last a lifetime. This chapter delves deep into building healthy habits by exploring techniques for integrating fitness into daily routines, overcoming common barriers, and the role of discipline and habit-forming in achieving long-term success.

Techniques to Integrate Fitness into Daily Routine

Integrating fitness into daily life may seem daunting initially, especially for individuals juggling demanding schedules, familial responsibilities, or career pressures. However, with the proper techniques, physical activity can seamlessly blend into everyday routines.

1. Prioritize Fitness in Your Schedule

- Treat fitness like any other commitment by blocking time for it on your calendar. This might involve setting aside 30 minutes in the morning or during a lunch break.
- Early mornings are ideal for workouts as they help set the tone for the day. Research suggests that exercising in the morning boosts energy levels and mental clarity.

2. Incorporate Physical Activity into Existing Habits

- Pair fitness activities with daily routines:
    - Use stairs instead of elevators.
    - Walk or bike to work or the store.
    - Stretch or do light exercises while watching TV.
- Habit stacking, a technique introduced by James Clear in *Atomic Habits*, suggests linking a new habit to an existing one. For example, do 10 squats after brushing your teeth.

3. Use Technology to Stay Accountable

- Fitness apps and wearable devices like Fitbit, Apple Watch, or Garmin can track your progress and send reminders.
- Online communities and fitness groups provide support and encouragement, fostering a sense of accountability.

4. Make Fitness Enjoyable

- Choose activities you genuinely enjoy. If you dislike running, try swimming, dancing, or cycling.
- Rotate activities to prevent monotony and target different muscle groups.

5. Incorporate Micro-Workouts

- Micro-workouts, or short bursts of exercise, are highly effective for busy schedules.
- For instance, 10-minute workouts throughout the day can accumulate into significant physical activity.

- Examples include desk push-ups, chair squats, or brisk walking between tasks.

6. Leverage Social Opportunities

- Turn fitness into a social activity by involving friends or family members.
- Join group classes, participate in community sports, or form walking groups in your neighborhood.

7. Focus on Functional Fitness

- Incorporate activities that mirror daily movements, such as lifting, bending, and reaching, to improve practical strength and reduce injury risk.

Strategies for Overcoming Common Barriers to Fitness

The journey to building healthy habits is often riddled with obstacles. Understanding and addressing these barriers is crucial to maintaining a consistent fitness routine.

1. Lack of Time

- Solution: Prioritize shorter, more intense workouts, such as high-intensity interval training (HIIT). Schedule workouts as non-negotiable appointments.
- Multitasking can help; for instance, take walking meetings or listen to audiobooks while jogging.

2. Lack of Motivation

- Solution: Set realistic and specific goals, such as losing 5 pounds in a month or completing a 5K race.
- Visualize the benefits of a healthier body, like improved energy, better sleep, or enhanced self-esteem.
- Reward yourself for milestones reached, but align rewards with your goals (e.g., buying new workout gear instead of indulging in unhealthy foods).

3. Cost Concerns

- Solution: Fitness doesn't have to be expensive. Bodyweight exercises, yoga, and running require minimal or no equipment.
- Explore free or low-cost resources like YouTube fitness channels, public parks, or community classes.

4. Physical Limitations or Health Issues

- Solution: Work with a healthcare provider or physical therapist to design a safe and effective exercise plan.
- Focus on low-impact activities such as swimming, walking, or chair exercises.

5. Fear of Judgment

- Solution: Start with at-home workouts until you feel more confident.

- Seek supportive environments like women-only gyms, beginner-friendly classes, or online communities.

6. Lack of Energy

- Solution: Adjust your diet and sleep schedule to optimize energy levels.
- Begin with light exercises, which boost energy over time.

7. Weather Constraints

- Solution: Have backup plans for inclement weather, such as indoor workouts or gym memberships.
- Use fitness apps to access guided exercises that don't require outdoor space.

The Role of Discipline and Habit-Forming in Long-Term Success

Discipline and habit formation are the cornerstones of sustained fitness and healthy living. While motivation can fluctuate, discipline ensures consistency.

1. Understand the Habit Loop Charles Duhigg, in The Power of Habit, describes the habit loop as consisting of three components:

- **Cue:** A trigger that initiates the habit. For instance, putting workout clothes by your bed can remind you to exercise in the morning.
- **Routine:** The behavior itself, such as exercising for 30 minutes.
- **Reward:** The benefit or pleasure derived from the habit, such as the endorphin rush after a workout.

By consciously designing this loop, you can replace unhealthy behaviors with positive ones.

2. Start Small and Build Gradually

- Begin with manageable goals. For instance, commit to exercising for 10 minutes daily instead of aiming for an hour.
- Gradual progress builds confidence and prevents burnout.

3. Establish a Consistent Routine

- Consistency is critical to forming habits. Exercising simultaneously each day helps embed the activity into your routine.
- Morning habits are particularly effective as they reduce the likelihood of procrastination.

4. Develop Mental Resilience

- Understand that setbacks are part of the journey. Missing a day or two doesn't mean failure—get back on track without guilt.
- Practice self-compassion and avoid all-or-nothing thinking.

5. Gamify the Process

- Turn fitness into a game by setting challenges, tracking streaks, or competing with friends.
- Use apps that reward milestones to keep you motivated.

6. Build a Support Network

- Share your goals with family or friends who can encourage and hold you accountable.
- Surround yourself with like-minded individuals to maintain a positive environment.

7. Focus on Identity Over Outcomes

- Shift your mindset from focusing solely on outcomes (e.g., losing 20 pounds) to embracing a new identity (e.g., becoming healthier).
- When fitness becomes a part of your identity, it's easier to sustain the habits.

8. Leverage Visualization and Positive Reinforcement

- Visualize your long-term goals and how achieving them will make you feel.
- Celebrate small wins to reinforce progress and keep momentum.

9. Utilize Habit Tracking

- Use journals or apps to track daily habits and review progress regularly.
- Seeing consistent streaks builds momentum and motivates continued effort.

10. Invest in Personal Development

- Read books or listen to podcasts on habit formation and personal growth.
- Continuous learning inspires innovation in your fitness journey.

Conclusion

Building healthy habits is a multi-faceted journey requiring clever techniques, perseverance, and self-awareness. Integrating fitness into your daily routine, overcoming common barriers, and focusing on discipline and habit formation can pave the way for a healthier and more fulfilling life. Remember, consistency is more important than perfection; every small step brings you closer to your goals.

Chapter 9: Nutrition Fundamentals

Nutrition is a cornerstone of health and physical performance. This chapter explores the essential principles of nutrition, the role of macronutrients, the connection between diet and physical activity, and practical strategies for designing a balanced diet tailored to fitness goals. Understanding these concepts is vital for anyone looking to improve their well-being and achieve specific physical performance outcomes.

1. **Basic Nutritional Concepts**

Nutrition refers to food intake and its impact on the body's health and function. The science of nutrition studies how various nutrients support growth, energy production, tissue repair, and overall homeostasis.

Critical Terms in Nutrition:

- **Nutrients:** Substances the body requires for energy, growth, and repair. They are categorized as macronutrients and micronutrients.
- **Caloric Balance:** The balance between calories consumed and expended. Maintaining, losing, or gaining weight depends on this balance.
- **Dietary Guidelines:** General recommendations for nutrient intake to promote health and reduce the risk of chronic diseases.

Macronutrients

Macronutrients provide the bulk of our energy and are required in large amounts. The three primary macronutrients are carbohydrates, proteins, and fats, each playing a distinct role in the body.

1.1 Carbohydrates

Carbohydrates are the body's primary energy source, especially for physical activity. They are broken down into glucose, which fuels the brain, muscles, and other tissues.

Types of Carbohydrates:

- **Simple Carbohydrates:** Quickly absorbed sugars, such as glucose and fructose, found in fruits, honey, and sweets.
- **Complex Carbohydrates:** Found in whole grains, vegetables, and legumes, these are digested slowly and provide sustained energy.

Benefits of Carbohydrates:

- The primary source of energy during high-intensity activities.
- Spare protein for its role in tissue repair and growth.
- Regulate blood sugar levels when consumed in their complex form.

Recommended Intake:

Carbohydrates should make up 45-65% of the daily caloric intake, depending on activity levels.

1.2 Proteins

Proteins are vital for building and repairing tissues, producing enzymes, and supporting immune function. They are made up of essential amino acids, some of which must be obtained from food.

Sources of Protein:

- **Complete Proteins:** Contains all essential amino acids found in animal products like meat, eggs, and dairy.
- **Incomplete Proteins:** Lack one or more essential amino acids, typically found in plant-based foods like beans and nuts.

Functions of Protein:

- Muscle repair and growth, especially after exercise.
- Hormone and enzyme production.
- Maintenance of immune health.

Recommended Intake:

Protein needs vary based on physical activity levels, ranging from 0.8 grams per kilogram of body weight for sedentary individuals to 1.2-2.0 grams for athletes.

1.3 Fats

Fats are a concentrated energy source, essential for nutrient absorption, hormone production, and cell membrane structure.

Types of Fats:

- **Saturated Fats,** found in animal products and some plant oils, can increase the risk of heart disease if consumed excessively.
- **Unsaturated Fats:** Healthy fats are found in nuts, seeds, fish, and avocados. They are further divided into monounsaturated and polyunsaturated fats.
- **Trans Fats:** Artificially hydrogenated fats that are harmful to health are found in processed foods.

Functions of Fats:

- Energy storage and insulation.
- Transport of fat-soluble vitamins (A, D, E, and K).
- Support for low-intensity, long-duration physical activities.

Recommended Intake:

Fats should constitute 20-35% of the daily caloric intake, with a focus on unsaturated fats.

1. **Relationship Between Diet and Physical Performance**

Nutrition and physical performance are interlinked, as proper fueling supports energy levels, recovery, and overall health.

2.1 Role of Carbohydrates in Performance

- Carbohydrates are the primary energy source for high-intensity workouts.
- Consuming carbs before exercise provides immediate energy, while post-exercise carbs replenish glycogen stores.

2.2 Importance of Protein for Recovery

- Protein aids muscle repair and synthesis post-exercise.

- A combination of protein and carbohydrates post-workout enhances glycogen replenishment and muscle recovery.

2.3 Fats and Sustained Energy

- Fats are the primary energy source during prolonged, moderate-intensity exercises like jogging or cycling.

- Athletes involved in endurance sports benefit from adequate fat intake.

2.4 Hydration and Performance

- Water is crucial for maintaining optimal performance, regulating body temperature, and preventing dehydration.

- Electrolyte balance is essential, particularly during extended workouts or in hot climates.

1. **Tips for Creating a Balanced Diet Supporting Fitness Goals**

A balanced diet ensures the right proportions of macronutrients and micronutrients to meet individual needs. Below are practical strategies for designing such a diet:

3.1 Establishing Caloric Needs

- Use Basal Metabolic Rate (BMR) calculators to determine daily caloric requirements based on age, sex, weight, and activity levels.

- Adjust caloric intake to match fitness goals—maintain, lose, or gain weight.

3.2 Macronutrient Distribution

- **For Weight Loss:** Focus on a high-protein, moderate-carb, low-fat diet to preserve muscle mass while reducing fat.

- **For Muscle Gain:** Increase protein and calorie intake with resistance training.

- **For Endurance Training:** Emphasize carbohydrates for sustained energy.

3.3 Meal Timing

- **Pre-Workout Meals:** Include easily digestible carbs and some protein to fuel workouts.
- **Post-Workout Meals:** Consume carbs and protein within 30 minutes to support recovery and muscle synthesis.

3.4 Incorporating Variety and Moderation

- Diversify food choices to ensure a range of nutrients.
- Practice moderation to prevent overconsumption of any one macronutrient.

3.5 Practical Meal Planning

- **Breakfast:** High in complex carbs (e.g., oats), moderate protein (e.g., eggs), and healthy fats (e.g., nuts).
- **Lunch:** Balanced meal with lean protein (e.g., chicken), whole grains (e.g., quinoa), and vegetables.
- **Snacks:** Nutritious options like fruits, yogurt, or trail mix.
- **Dinner:** Lighter on carbs, higher in protein and vegetables.

3.6 Supplements

- Consider supplements like whey protein or multivitamins if dietary intake is insufficient.
- Always consult a healthcare provider before adding supplements.

1. **Final Thoughts**

Achieving fitness goals requires a strong understanding of nutritional fundamentals. Tailoring macronutrient intake and meal timing to individual needs can optimize physical performance and overall health. Focusing on a balanced, nutrient-dense diet ensures long-term success and sustainability in health and fitness pursuits.

Chapter 10: Dispelling Fitness Myths

Introduction to Fitness Myths

- **Importance of debunking myths**: In the information age, fitness myths are rampant, often fueled by anecdotal evidence, misleading advertisements, or outdated scientific theories. This chapter challenges these misconceptions and provides evidence-based insights to guide people toward healthier, more effective fitness practices.

1. **Common Misconceptions About Fitness and Exercise**
2. **Myth: "You need to work out daily to see results."**
   - **Reality**: Rest is crucial for muscle recovery and overall health. Overtraining without adequate rest can lead to fatigue, injuries, and decreased performance.
   - **Scientific Insight**: Studies show that muscles need at least 24-48 hours of recovery time after a strength training session for optimal repair and growth. Consistent rest days allow the body to rebuild, grow, and adapt.
3. **Myth: "No pain, no gain."**
   - **Reality**: While challenging workouts may result in discomfort or soreness, pain (exceptionally sharp or acute) is a sign of injury, not progress.
   - **Scientific Insight**: Research on muscle soreness (DOMS – delayed onset muscle soreness) reveals that while it's common after intense workouts, pain does not correlate with muscle growth or strength. Pushing through pain can lead to injury.
4. **Myth: "Cardio is the best way to lose fat."**
   - **Reality**: While cardio (such as running, cycling, or swimming) effectively burns calories, fat loss is primarily driven by creating a caloric deficit. This can be achieved through both diet and exercise, including strength training.
   - **Scientific Insight**: Strength training has been shown to increase lean muscle mass, which in turn boosts metabolism and helps the body burn more calories at rest. Combining cardio with strength training often produces superior fat-loss results.
5. **Myth: "You can spot-reduce fat."**
   - **Reality**: Targeting specific body areas for fat loss through exercises like abdominal crunches or thigh lifts is a myth. Fat loss occurs across the whole body based on genetics and caloric deficit.

- **Scientific Insight**: Studies have shown that spot-reduction is not possible. When you lose weight, it happens throughout your entire body, not just in the area you're exercising. Overall, fat loss is best achieved through diet and exercise.

6. **Myth: "Strength training makes women bulky."**
    - **Reality**: Strength training will not make women "bulky" unless they intentionally aim to gain significant muscle mass through heavy lifting and specific dietary plans.
    - **Scientific Insight**: Women have lower levels of testosterone than men, making it harder for them to gain large amounts of muscle. Strength training, especially with moderate weight and higher reps, helps women build lean muscle, which enhances metabolism, posture, and overall body composition.

7. **Myth: "Lifting heavy weights is dangerous."**
    - **Reality**: Lifting heavy weights is not inherently dangerous when performed with proper technique. Strength training is one of the most effective ways to build bone density, increase muscle mass, and improve overall functional strength.
    - **Scientific Insight**: Research has shown that weight lifting is safe and beneficial with the correct form and progressive overload. It improves cardiovascular health, boosts metabolism, and prevents age-related muscle loss.

8. **Scientific Evidence Debunking Popular Fitness Myths**

9. **The Myth of "The Fat Burning Zone" in Cardio:**
    - **Reality**: Many people believe that exercising at a lower intensity (e.g., walking or light jogging) burns fatter due to the concept of the "fat-burning zone." However, higher-intensity exercise burns more calories overall, including fat.
    - **Scientific Insight**: Lower-intensity exercise may burn a higher percentage of fat during the workout, but higher-intensity exercises (such as HIIT or sprinting) burn more total calories and fat in the long run. Studies show that post-workout fat burn (EPOC – Excess Post-Exercise Oxygen Consumption) is elevated after high-intensity exercise.

10. **The Myth of "Eating Fat Makes You Fat":**
    - **Reality**: Fat is an essential nutrient, and dietary fats (when consumed in healthy forms) do not directly contribute to fat

gain. Overeating calories, regardless of the macronutrient source, leads to fat gain.

- **Scientific Insight**: Research has shown that fat is necessary for hormone regulation, brain function, and cellular health. Healthy fats, such as those from avocados, nuts, and fish, are crucial for overall health and do not inherently lead to weight gain when consumed in moderation.

11. **The Myth of "Carbs Make You Fat":**
    - **Reality**: Carbohydrates are the body's preferred energy source, especially during high-intensity exercise. It's not carbs that make you fat, but excessive calorie intake.
    - **Scientific Insight**: The body uses carbohydrates for energy, and cutting them out entirely can negatively impact athletic performance and recovery. Research indicates that a balanced intake of complex carbs supports sustainable energy levels and recovery from exercise.

12. **The Myth of "You Need Supplements to Build Muscle."**
    - **Reality**: While certain supplements may support performance and recovery, they are not magic solutions for muscle growth. A well-rounded diet and consistent exercise are the most critical factors.
    - **Scientific Insight**: Creatine, protein powders, and branched-chain amino acids (BCAAs) are among the most researched and supported supplements for muscle gain. However, they must find a way to replace the fundamental need for a balanced diet and progressive resistance training.

13. **The Myth of "Women Should Avoid Heavy Lifting."**
    - **Reality**: The idea that women should avoid heavy lifting because it will make them "too muscular" is a persistent myth. Strength training benefits women of any age and is crucial for health, fat loss, and muscle tone.
    - **Scientific Insight**: Strength training enhances muscle mass, boosts metabolism, and protects bone health. Women in strength training benefit from improved muscle endurance, functional strength, and cardiovascular health.

14. **Encouraging Critical Thinking and Research in Fitness**

15. **Be Skeptical of "Quick Fix" Solutions:**
    - **Reality**: Fitness is a long-term journey that requires commitment, proper education, and consistent effort. Be wary of advertisements promising rapid results or "secret" methods for instant transformation.

- **Research Tip**: When researching fitness topics, always look for credible sources such as peer-reviewed studies, reputable fitness organizations (like the American College of Sports Medicine), and certified fitness professionals.

16. **The Importance of Evidence-Based Fitness Practices:**
    - **Reality**: Research-backed fitness practices are more reliable than anecdotal advice. For example, resistance training and progressive overload have been scientifically proven effective for building strength and muscle.
    - **Scientific Insight**: Look for studies published in well-known sports science journals to verify claims. Peer-reviewed studies that use control groups and measure long-term outcomes are the most reliable indicators of what works in fitness.

17. **Questioning Trends and Fads:**
    - **Reality**: A new fitness trend emerges every few years, promising miraculous results with minimal effort. It's essential to approach such trends with a healthy skepticism and research before adopting them.
    - **Example**: Fad diets like keto, intermittent fasting, or juice may have some benefits for specific individuals, but they are not universally effective and often have long-term health risks if not properly implemented.

18. **The Role of Personalization in Fitness:**
    - **Reality**: Fitness is not one-size-fits-all. Individual factors such as age, genetics, fitness level, and goals significantly determine the best fitness approach for you.

- **Scientific Insight**: Research indicates that tailored fitness programs based on personal goals (fat loss, muscle gain, endurance, etc.) yield better results than generic "one-size-fits-all" plans.

Conclusion: Promoting a Healthier, More Informed Approach to Fitness

- **The Path Forward**: In a world filled with misinformation, the key to achieving lasting fitness goals is understanding the science behind exercise and nutrition. By dispelling myths, staying informed, and being critical of unproven claims, individuals can pursue fitness in a sustainable, healthy, and effective way.

- **Action Steps for Readers**:
  - Question myths and educate yourself through reputable sources.
  - Focus on the long-term benefits of exercise rather than chasing instant results.
  - Find a workout routine that suits your body and lifestyle, and remember that consistency is critical.

Conclusion

1. This chapter highlights the importance of critical thinking when approaching fitness advice. Debunking popular myths allows readers to avoid harmful or ineffective practices and embrace scientifically-backed methods for achieving fitness goals. Through continued research and an open mind, individuals can build a fitness routine tailored to their needs, ensuring long-term success and well-being.

Chapter 11: Motivation and Mindset

Introduction

The chapter focuses on the psychological aspects of maintaining a fitness routine, building mental resilience, and fostering a growth mindset to overcome setbacks. It acknowledges that fitness is not just a physical endeavor but also requires mental fortitude and a positive attitude. Understanding how motivation works, what influences our ability to stay committed, and how to manage setbacks is crucial for achieving long-term fitness success.

Psychological Aspects of Maintaining a Fitness Routine

Maintaining a fitness routine is often more challenging than it seems on paper. It involves a combination of physical effort, time management, and, above all, mental discipline. Psychology plays a significant role in whether or not individuals can stick to a fitness regimen.

1. **Intrinsic vs. Extrinsic Motivation:** Motivation can be divided into intrinsic (internal) and extrinsic (external) forms. Intrinsic motivation comes from within, such as the joy of achieving personal goals or the satisfaction of personal growth. On the other hand, extrinsic motivation involves external rewards, such as praise, recognition, or tangible rewards (e.g., a new pair of running shoes). Studies suggest intrinsic motivation leads to more sustainable and long-term engagement with fitness routines.

   - **Intrinsic Motivation Example**: Feeling better physically and mentally after a workout.
   - **Extrinsic Motivation Example**: A reward system where you treat yourself to something special after reaching a fitness goal.

2. **Habits and Routine Formation:** Psychological research suggests that forming new habits relies on consistency. In the case of fitness, consistency is crucial. Integrating fitness into daily routines becomes part of your identity rather than something you "have to do." This gradual shift in mindset can help individuals maintain a regular fitness regimen, even when motivation is low.

3. **The Role of Willpower:** Willpower plays a central role in adhering to fitness plans. It's what helps people push through moments of fatigue, discomfort, or boredom. However, willpower is finite; it can be depleted over time. Developing other strategies, such as creating a schedule or having a workout buddy, is essential to support the fitness routine without over-relying on willpower alone.

4. **The Power of Mental Imagery:** Visualization is a technique athletes and fitness enthusiasts use to enhance performance. Individuals mentally rehearsing workouts or picturing success can train their brains to anticipate success and improve motivation. Imagery can also be used to focus on the physical and emotional benefits of exercising, helping to strengthen the desire to continue.

Techniques for Building Mental Resilience and Motivation

Mental resilience is the ability to recover from setbacks, adapt to challenges, and keep moving forward. In the context of fitness, it is the quality that enables individuals to push through obstacles and continue pursuing their goals despite challenges.

1. **Goal Setting:** Setting clear, achievable goals is one of the most effective ways to maintain motivation. The goals should be:
   - **Specific**: Define what you want to achieve.
   - **Measurable**: Include metrics that track progress.
   - **Achievable**: Set realistic expectations that are still challenging.
   - **Relevant**: Ensure that goals are aligned with your overall fitness journey.
   - **Time-bound**: Have a deadline to keep yourself accountable.

2. Goals can be short-term (e.g., attending the gym three times a week) and long-term (e.g., completing a marathon). The sense of accomplishment from reaching these goals helps maintain motivation.

3. **The Power of Positive Self-Talk:** Negative self-talk can significantly hinder progress. Phrases like "I'm too tired to work out" or "I'll never reach my goal" can undermine motivation. In contrast, positive self-talk can help to reframe challenges and boost self-confidence. For example, instead of thinking, "I can't do this," you might say, "I've faced tough workouts before and succeeded."
   - **Affirmations**: Repeating positive affirmations can help reprogram your mindset. For instance, saying "I am strong and capable" can shift focus from doubts to confidence.

4. **Building a Support System:** A support system is essential for maintaining motivation and mental resilience. This can be through workout buddies, a personal trainer, online fitness communities, or friends and family who encourage you. A social network not only provides accountability but can also inspire you with their own success stories, creating a sense of camaraderie.

5. **Managing Stress and Anxiety:** Stress, anxiety, or overwhelming emotions can sometimes disrupt fitness routines. Learning to manage these psychological states is essential for mental resilience. Techniques such as mindfulness, deep breathing, meditation, or even taking a break can help alleviate stress and prevent it from affecting your fitness routine.

6. **Celebrate Small Wins:** Recognizing and celebrating small victories, such as improving your stamina or lifting heavier weights, can fuel motivation. Acknowledging progress, even if it's not directly tied to the final goal, helps to reinforce the habit of consistency and reminds individuals that their efforts are paying off.

7. **Self-Compassion:** Being kind to oneself during tough times is critical for mental resilience. Fitness journeys are not linear, and setbacks are natural. When you miss a workout or fall short of a goal,

practicing self-compassion helps to avoid negative self-criticism, which can demotivate and lead to giving up. Instead of saying, "I failed," reframe it as "I'll do better next time."

Importance of a Growth Mindset in Overcoming Setbacks

The growth mindset concept, developed by psychologist Carol Dweck, posits that intelligence and abilities are not fixed traits but can be developed with effort, learning, and perseverance. A growth mindset is essential for overcoming setbacks in life, including fitness.

1. **Fixed vs. Growth Mindset:**

    - **Fixed Mindset**: Believing that your abilities are static and cannot be improved. Individuals with a fixed mindset may give up easily after encountering challenges, as they view failure as a sign of inability.

    - **Growth Mindset**: Believing that challenges are growth opportunities. Those with a growth mindset understand that failure is part of the learning process and that persistence can lead to eventual success.

2. In fitness, individuals with a growth mindset view setbacks as part of the journey. For example, missing a personal best during a workout is a temporary hurdle rather than a permanent roadblock.

3. **Overcoming Setbacks with Resilience:** The growth mindset encourages individuals to see obstacles not as insurmountable challenges but as opportunities to learn and improve. When setbacks occur, such as an injury or a plateau in performance, the growth mindset prompts individuals to seek solutions, adjust their approach, and continue moving forward.

    - **Example:** If a runner injures their leg, someone with a growth mindset might see this as an opportunity to focus on upper body strength or work on flexibility while recovering rather than abandoning fitness altogether.

4. **Embracing Challenges:** A growth mindset fosters a willingness to take on challenges that might initially seem intimidating. This could involve trying new exercises, attempting more challenging workout routines, or participating in a fitness competition. When challenges are viewed as opportunities for growth, individuals are more likely to take risks and push their limits.

5. **Learning from Failure:** Failure is inevitable in fitness, as in any other area. Whether failing to achieve a goal or not performing well on a particular day, how we respond to failure makes all the difference. Those with a growth mindset learn from their failures by asking themselves questions like "What can I do differently next time?" or "How can I improve?"

6. **Persistence and Effort:** A vital aspect of the growth mindset is the belief that effort leads to improvement. In fitness, this translates to the understanding that progress comes with consistent hard work and dedication, even if results are not immediately visible. Individuals with a growth mindset are more likely to persist through tough times because they believe their efforts will eventually pay off.

Conclusion

In conclusion, psychological factors such as motivation, mental resilience, and a growth mindset are critical to a successful fitness routine. Individuals can overcome challenges by cultivating intrinsic motivation, setting clear goals, building resilience, adopting a growth mindset, and staying committed to their fitness journeys. Mental strength is just as important as physical ability, and by understanding and applying psychological strategies, individuals can make fitness a lifelong habit.

Chapter 12: Tracking Your Progress

Tracking your fitness progress is one of the most important aspects of maintaining motivation, ensuring an effective training plan, and achieving long-term fitness goals. Without tracking, it can be difficult to see how far you've come or identify areas where adjustments may be needed. In this chapter, we explore the tools and methods for monitoring progress, how to recognize and celebrate improvements, and how to make necessary adjustments to your plans based on feedback and results.

1. **Tools and Methods for Monitoring Fitness Progress**

Monitoring progress is essential for understanding the effectiveness of your fitness routine and making informed decisions moving forward. Various tools and methods are available to track fitness progress, ranging from high-tech gadgets to simple manual tracking. These tools can help assess multiple aspects of fitness, such as strength, endurance, flexibility, and body composition. Below are some of the most commonly used tools and methods:

1.1. Fitness Trackers and Wearables

Fitness trackers, such as smartwatches (e.g., Apple Watch, Fitbit, Garmin), are one of the most popular tools for tracking physical activity and progress. These devices can monitor a wide range of metrics, including:

- **Heart rate:** To assess cardiovascular fitness.
- **Step count:** Monitor daily activity levels and encourage a more active lifestyle.
- **Calories burned:** To estimate energy expenditure, essential for weight management.
- **Sleep patterns:** Quality of sleep can significantly impact recovery and overall performance.
- **Distance and speed:** Particularly useful for runners, cyclists, and other endurance athletes.

Many trackers sync with mobile apps, providing a detailed breakdown of daily, weekly, and monthly activity levels.

1.2. Mobile Apps for Fitness Tracking

Several mobile applications are designed to help you track different aspects of your fitness journey. These apps can track workouts, nutrition, and progress over time. Some examples include:

- **MyFitnessPal:** Popular for monitoring food intake and macronutrients.
- **Strava:** Ideal for tracking running, cycling, and other endurance activities.
- **Nike Training Club:** A comprehensive app for guided workouts that can be customized to individual goals.
- **Strong Lifts 5x5:** Designed specifically for strength training and tracking workout progress in weightlifting. These apps allow you to set goals, monitor daily progress, and track specific performance metrics (e.g., reps, sets, weight lifted, or miles run).

1.3. Fitness Assessments

Fitness assessments are a more structured way to track progress and provide baseline measurements for your fitness journey. Common assessments include:

- **Body Composition Analysis** includes measuring body fat percentage and muscle mass. Tools like skinfold calipers, bioelectrical impedance scales, and DEXA scans can provide insights into how your body changes over time.
- **VO2 Max Testing:** VO2 Max measures your aerobic capacity or the maximum amount of oxygen your body can utilize during intense exercise. It's often used to assess cardiovascular fitness.
- **Strength Assessments:** Recording the maximum weight you can lift for a given number of reps (e.g., one-rep max) or tracking your improvement over time (e.g., lifting heavier weights or doing more reps) is a reliable indicator of strength progress.
- **Flexibility Testing:** Stretching assessments, like the sit-and-reach test, can evaluate flexibility and track improvements.
- **Endurance Tests:** The Cooper Test (running as far as possible in 12 minutes) or timed mile runs are examples of endurance assessments that track cardiovascular fitness and stamina.

1.4. Journaling and Manual Tracking

For some people, journaling is the most effective way to track progress. Writing down daily or weekly logs of workouts, nutrition, mood, and sleep patterns can provide valuable insights. This can be done either in a physical notebook or digitally using apps or spreadsheets. Tracking variables such as:

- **Exercise type and duration**
- **Sets, reps, and weights lifted**
- **Diet and nutrition**
- **Rest and recovery times**
- **Mood or energy levels**

Regularly reviewing your journal entries allows you to observe trends and make adjustments as necessary. This method can also help identify any patterns that need to be addressed, such as plateaus or dips in performance.

1.5. Progress Photos

Taking regular progress photos is a visual tool that helps you see the physical changes in your body. Often, people can't notice subtle changes daily, but the transformation can become much more apparent when comparing photos over weeks or months. This can be motivating, especially for those focused on fat loss or muscle gain.

1.6. Performance-Based Metrics

In addition to physical measures, tracking performance milestones can provide valuable feedback on progress. These might include:

- **Personal bests (PBs):** These could be lifting heavier weights, running faster, or performing more reps in a given exercise.
- **Skill development:** Progress might be seen in mastering new exercises or techniques, such as achieving a pull-up or improving your form on squats or deadlifts.
1. **Recognizing and Celebrating Improvements**

Recognizing progress and celebrating improvements is crucial for maintaining motivation and staying committed to your fitness goals. It's easy to become discouraged when focusing on the end goal rather than acknowledging the smaller milestones. Here are some strategies to help you celebrate progress:

2.1. Small Wins Lead to Big Gains

Fitness is a long-term journey; small wins often lead to more considerable successes. These small wins can include:

- **Increased strength:** Lifting heavier weights or completing more reps.
- **Endurance improvements:** Running longer distances or cycling at faster speeds.
- **Consistency:** Sticking to your workout schedule for a certain period.
- **Body composition changes** A reduced body fat percentage or increased lean muscle mass.

These small wins should be celebrated through an internal acknowledgment or a reward, such as treating yourself to a massage, a new workout outfit, or a favorite healthy meal.

2.2. Focus on Non-Squale Victoires (NS Vs)

While weight loss is often a primary goal for many, focusing on non-scale victories (NSVs) is also essential. These victories might include:

- **Improved energy levels** throughout the day.
- **Better sleep quality** and rest.
- **Increased strength** and stamina.
- **Improved mental health**, such as reduced stress or anxiety.
- **Increased confidence** and body positivity. NSVs often provide more significant and sustainable motivation than simply watching the number on the scale fluctuate.

2.3. Share Your Successes with Others

Sharing your fitness achievements with friends, family, or a fitness community can be highly motivating. Celebrating with others reinforces your sense of accomplishment and inspires those around you to take their fitness journey seriously.

2.4. Positive Self-Talk

Acknowledge your progress through positive self-talk. Celebrate what you have accomplished instead of focusing on what you haven't achieved. Recognize that even if you haven't reached your ultimate goal, you are still making progress, which is worth celebrating.

1. **Adjusting Plans Based on Feedback and Results**

Tracking your progress provides critical feedback that can guide necessary adjustments to your fitness plan. Regular adjustments based on this feedback help prevent plateaus, overtraining, or injury and ensure you always progress toward your goals. Here are some common ways to adjust your plan:

3.1. Modifying Workout Intensity

As you progress, your body adapts to the stress you place on it. If you don't increase the intensity of your workouts over time, you'll hit a plateau. To continue progressing, you may need to:

- **Increase the resistance:** Lift heavier weights or add more resistance to exercises.
- **Change the volume:** Perform more sets or reps for a particular exercise.
- **Alter workout frequency:** Add an extra workout day per week or incorporate additional sets or circuits into your existing routine.
- **Include progressive overload:** Continuously challenge your body by gradually sustainably increasing intensity.

3.2. Rest and Recovery Adjustments

If you notice a lack of progress, fatigue, or soreness that doesn't seem to subside, it may be a sign that you're overtraining and need to adjust your recovery. Overtraining can lead to injuries and burnout. Ensuring proper rest and recovery can involve:

- **Increased rest days** to allow your muscles to repair and grow.
- **Active recovery** (e.g., walking, yoga, light swimming) on non-training days.
- **Sleep optimization** to promote muscle recovery.
- **Proper nutrition** with a focus on protein intake to support muscle repair.

3.3. Diet and Nutrition Tweaks

Nutrition plays a massive role in supporting fitness goals. Consider adjusting your diet if you're still waiting to see your expected progress. For example:

- **Caloric intake:** Ensure you're eating enough calories to fuel your workouts or adjust if you're trying to lose weight.
- **Macronutrient balance:** If strength training is your priority, ensure you consume enough protein to build muscle.
- **Meal timing:** Consider nutrient timing, such as eating protein before or after a workout for muscle recovery.

3.4. Changing Your Routine

If you've been doing the same workout for weeks or months, your body may stop responding. This is known as the principle of "specificity." To keep making progress, vary your routine by:

- **Incorporating new exercises** or workout

Chapter 13: Importance of Rest and Recovery

1. Understanding the Role of Rest in Fitness

Rest is an often-underestimated aspect of fitness training. Many athletes and fitness enthusiasts focus solely on physical activity—lifting weights, running, cycling, or engaging in high-intensity workouts—while ignoring the importance of rest. However, rest plays a critical role in the body's ability to recover, repair, and improve performance. Rest isn't just about taking a break; it is an active process contributing to physical and mental well-being.

Physiological Recovery Mechanisms

When you engage in physical exercise, particularly resistance training or endurance activities, your body experiences stress. This stress causes microtears in muscle fibers, which leads to soreness and fatigue. The recovery process involves repairing and rebuilding these muscle fibers, resulting in increased muscle strength, endurance, and overall performance. Without sufficient rest, the body does not have adequate time to heal these microtears, which can hinder progress and lead to overtraining.

In addition to muscular recovery, the cardiovascular, nervous, and hormonal systems all require rest to recover from intense physical activity. For example, the body needs time to replenish glycogen stores, reduce inflammation, and restore hormonal balance. Cortisol (the stress hormone) levels rise during exercise, and the body needs to return to baseline through proper rest, ensuring the body's natural recovery mechanisms are functioning effectively.

Rest and Performance Enhancement

The key to progress in fitness is not simply the amount of exercise but the balance between training and recovery. Over time, with consistent exercise followed by adequate rest, the body adapts, becoming more resilient, robust, and capable of handling more significant physical stress. If you neglect recovery, you can experience a plateau in performance or, worse, a decline in fitness levels. Performance improvements are typically seen during the recovery period, where the body rebuilds muscle tissue and adapts to the stress placed on it.

Moreover, mental recovery is equally important. Intense training regimens can lead to mental fatigue and reduced motivation. Rest and recovery allow the body to recover physically and give the mind a chance to reset, which is essential for maintaining motivation and enthusiasm for future workouts.

1. Different Recovery Techniques and Practices

Recovery is a multifaceted process involving several strategies to ensure physical and mental rejuvenation. Here are some of the most effective recovery techniques:

Active Recovery

Active recovery involves engaging in low-intensity exercise after intense workouts. It helps maintain blood circulation, which in turn aids in removing metabolic waste products like lactic acid that accumulate during intense training. Active recovery activities include:

- **Light jogging or cycling** – Keeps the heart rate elevated without causing further strain on the muscles.
- **Swimming** – The buoyancy of water supports the body, reducing joint stress while allowing for full-body movement.
- **Yoga or stretching** – Gentle stretching and yoga help release muscle tension and improve flexibility, contributing to relaxation and recovery.

Active recovery has been shown to reduce soreness, promote flexibility, and speed up muscle repair.

Passive Recovery

Passive recovery is rest without any physical activity. This can include activities such as:

- **Sleep** – Sleep is one of the most critical elements in any recovery regimen. During sleep, the body releases growth hormones, rebuilds tissue, and replenishes energy stores. Aim for 7-9 hours of sleep per night to support optimal recovery.
- **Rest days** – Designated days where no physical activity is performed. These days, it is essential to allow muscles to be fully repaired and to prevent the risk of overtraining.
- **Massage therapy** – A deep tissue massage or foam rolling can help reduce muscle tension, improve circulation, and speed recovery.

While passive recovery does not involve active movement, it is essential for providing the body with complete respite and the opportunity to repair damaged tissues.

Nutrition and Hydration

Proper nutrition plays an essential role in the recovery process. After exercise, the body requires nutrients to repair muscle fibers, replenish glycogen stores, and reduce inflammation. A balanced post-workout meal that includes protein, carbohydrates, and fats can facilitate optimal recovery.

- **Protein** – Essential for muscle repair and recovery. Consuming protein-rich foods like chicken, fish, eggs, or plant-based protein sources is recommended within an hour after exercise.
- **Carbohydrates** – Carbs help replenish glycogen stores that are depleted during prolonged or intense exercise. Fruits, whole grains, and starchy vegetables are good carbohydrate sources.
- **Fats** – Healthy fats support joint health and provide energy. Omega-3 fatty acids found in fish oil, flaxseeds, and walnuts are particularly beneficial for reducing inflammation.

- **Hydration** – Proper hydration is crucial to recovery. Water helps transport nutrients to muscles and flush out toxins. During intense workouts, it is also essential to replenish lost electrolytes through sports drinks or coconut water.

Fueling the body with the proper nutrients and staying hydrated provides the energy required for muscle repair and overall recovery.

Cold and Heat Therapy

Both cold and heat therapies have been used for centuries to enhance recovery, though their application depends on the nature of the injury or soreness.

- **Cold Therapy (Cryotherapy)** – Cold therapy, such as ice baths or cold compresses, helps reduce inflammation and numb pain. It is instrumental in the immediate aftermath of an intense workout or injury.
- **Heat Therapy** – Heat therapy, such as hot tubs or heating pads, can increase muscle blood flow, helping heal. It is beneficial for chronic muscle tightness and stiffness.

Many athletes alternate between hot and cold treatments in **contrast therapy**, where they alternate between hot and cold to stimulate circulation and reduce inflammation.

Compression Therapy

Compression garments or devices, such as compression socks or sleeves, can help reduce swelling and muscle soreness. These garments provide constant pressure, improving circulation and reducing lactic acid buildup in muscles. While the evidence is mixed, many athletes report feeling fresher and less sore after using compression therapy.

Mindfulness and Stress Management

Mental recovery is just as important as physical recovery. Stress can impair the body's ability to recover from physical exertion, so managing mental health through relaxation techniques is essential. Meditation, **deep breathing, progressive muscle relaxation,** and **mindfulness** can lower cortisol levels, improve sleep quality, and enhance overall well-being. Reducing stress also promotes a better mental attitude toward future workouts.

1. **Preventing Burnout and Overtraining**

While regular exercise is essential for physical and mental health, too much exercise without adequate rest can lead to burnout or overtraining. Overtraining syndrome (OTS) occurs when an athlete or fitness enthusiast pushes the body beyond its capacity to recover, leading to a decline in performance and a range of physical and psychological symptoms.

Signs and Symptoms of Overtraining

Overtraining can manifest in both physical and psychological symptoms, including:

- **Fatigue** – Persistent tiredness that does not improve with rest.
- **Decreased performance** – A noticeable decline in strength, endurance, or overall performance.
- **Mood disturbances** – Increased irritability, anxiety, or depression.
- **Increased injury risk** – More frequent strains, sprains, or other injuries due to inadequate recovery.
- **Insomnia or poor sleep quality** – Difficulty falling asleep or staying asleep due to excessive training.
- **Decreased appetite** – Loss of interest in food or gastrointestinal issues.

If left unchecked, overtraining can lead to more severe health issues, such as immune system dysfunction or hormonal imbalances.

Preventing Overtraining

To prevent overtraining and burnout, listening to your body and implementing proper recovery strategies is essential. Here are some tips:

- **Schedule Rest Days** – Plan regular rest days and avoid training on consecutive days, especially if you're doing high-intensity workouts.
- **Monitor Training Load** – Gradually increase the intensity and volume of your training. Avoid sudden spikes in exercise that can overwhelm the body.
- **Ensure Proper Sleep** – Aim for sufficient sleep each night to allow the body to recover fully.
- **Use a Balanced Approach** – Combine different types of exercise (strength, cardiovascular, flexibility) and alternate between high and low-intensity workouts.
- **Cross-Training** – Vary your activities to prevent burnout. For instance, if you're a runner, try swimming or cycling to give your legs a break.
- **Nutrition and Hydration** – Fuel your body with the proper nutrients and stay hydrated to aid recovery and prevent fatigue.

Conclusion

Rest and recovery are vital components of any fitness regimen. They allow the body and mind to repair, rejuvenate, and adapt to the stresses during exercise. Incorporating effective recovery practices into your routine enhances performance and reduces the risk of burnout, overtraining, and injury. By understanding the importance of rest, applying various recovery techniques, and listening to your body's needs, you can optimize your fitness results and maintain a balanced, healthy lifestyle.

Chapter 14: Equipment and Gear Guide

Introduction:

Whether done at home or in the gym, fitness training requires the right equipment to ensure effectiveness, safety, and convenience. For beginners, navigating the vast world of fitness gear can be overwhelming. This chapter aims to demystify choosing and using fitness equipment, helping readers make informed decisions based on their goals, space, and budget. Whether you are just starting or looking to upgrade your gear, this guide will provide valuable insights into selecting the right equipment for your workouts.

1. **Overview of Essential Fitness Equipment for Beginners**

For beginners, starting with the right fitness equipment is crucial to ensure a smooth and effective journey into fitness. The most essential equipment doesn't necessarily mean expensive or high-tech gear. Many beginners can achieve great results with crucial, affordable equipment.

a. Resistance Bands: Resistance bands are among the most versatile and inexpensive tools for beginners. They can target nearly every muscle group and are especially useful for strength training exercises. Their adjustable resistance levels suit both novices and more advanced fitness enthusiasts.

- **Benefits:**
    - They are great for beginners as they provide controlled resistance.
    - It can be used for full-body workouts or isolated muscle groups.
    - Portable and ideal for home workouts or travel.

b. Dumbbells: Dumbbells are another staple of strength training. Beginners should start with light weights to perfect their form and avoid injury. Dumbbells come in a variety of weights, allowing progression as strength improves.

- **Benefits:**
    - Effective for building muscle and enhancing endurance.
    - Suitable for various exercises, including bicep curls, shoulder presses, and squats.
    - Compact and easy to store.

c. Stability Ball: A stability ball (a Swiss ball) is used for balance exercises, core training, and flexibility routines. It helps improve coordination, posture, and stability.

- **Benefits:**
    - Engages the core muscles while performing exercises.
    - Versatile—can be used for various exercises, including sit-ups, squats, and stretches.
    - Encourages correct posture and body alignment.

d. Kettlebells: Kettlebells are a unique form of weight training equipment designed to improve strength and cardiovascular fitness through dynamic, full-body movements.

- **Benefits:**
    - Ideal for functional fitness and full-body workouts.
    - It can improve both strength and endurance.

- Compact, allowing for easy storage and versatile use at home or in a gym.

e. Jump Rope: A jump rope is an inexpensive and effective cardiovascular workout tool that also helps improve coordination, timing, and agility.

- **Benefits:**
  - Great for full-body cardiovascular conditioning.
  - Portable and can be used in small spaces.
  - Enhances footwork, endurance, and muscle tone.

f. Foam Roller: A foam roller is essential for muscle recovery. It helps release muscle tension, improve flexibility, and reduce soreness.

- **Benefits:**
  - Aids in self-myofascial release to alleviate tight muscles.
  - Reduces post-workout soreness and enhances flexibility.
  - Easy to use after workouts for muscle recovery.

g. Yoga Mat: A yoga mat is essential for those interested in yoga, Pilates, or stretching. It provides a non-slip surface for floor exercises and can help prevent injuries during stretching or relaxation routines.

- **Benefits:**
  - Provides comfort and stability during bodyweight exercises.
  - Essential for floor-based workouts.
  - Lightweight and easy to store.

h. Treadmill/Stationary Bike (Optional for Home Gyms): Cardio equipment like a treadmill or stationary bike is useful for beginners who prefer to do aerobic exercises at home rather than go to a gym.

- **Benefits:**
  - Allows you to perform low-impact cardiovascular exercise in the comfort of your home.
  - It can be adjusted for different fitness levels.
  - Helps with weight loss, endurance, and overall cardiovascular health.

1. **Tips on Choosing the Right Gear for Various Workouts**

Choosing the right fitness gear largely depends on the type of workout you plan to do. Below are some key considerations and tips for selecting the appropriate equipment for different fitness routines.

a. Strength Training:

- **Start Simple:** If you're new to weightlifting, begin with essential equipment like dumbbells, resistance bands, and kettlebells. Once you master these, you can gradually incorporate heavier equipment, like barbells or specialized machines.
- **Form Over Weight:** Focus on using light weights initially to perfect your form before increasing the weight load.
- **Adjustable Gear:** Consider adjustable dumbbells or kettlebells, as they allow you to increase or decrease the weight according to your workout intensity.

b. Cardiovascular Workouts:

- **Footwear:** Proper shoes are crucial for running or walking to prevent injury. Choose shoes with proper arch support and cushioning.

- **Home Cardio:** If space or budget are limited, a jump rope or compact stationary bike are excellent options. For those with more space, a treadmill or elliptical machine can be ideal for longer cardio sessions.
- **Outdoor Cardio:** If you prefer outdoor activities like running or cycling, invest in a high-quality pair of running shoes or a reliable bicycle suited to your outdoor terrain.

c. Flexibility and Balance Workouts:

- **Yoga & Pilates:** A yoga mat is essential for floor-based exercises. If you practice yoga regularly, consider purchasing blocks and straps to deepen your stretches and improve flexibility.
- **Stability Balls & Bands:** These tools benefit balance and stability exercises, enhancing core strength and posture.

d. Functional Training:

- **Functional Training Gear:** Dumbbells, kettlebells, and resistance bands are highly effective for functional movements (e.g., squats, lunges, deadlifts). These tools mimic real-life movements, improving strength and mobility.
- **Adjustable Bench:** An adjustable bench is an excellent investment for beginners looking to perform exercises like dumbbell presses, chest flies, and incline/decline presses.

1. **Recommendations for Home vs. Gym Settings**

a. Home Gym Recommendations:

For those with limited space or a preference for working out at home, choosing equipment that offers versatility and can be stored easily is essential.

- **Compact Gear:** Resistance bands, dumbbells, kettlebells, and jump ropes take up little space and can be used for various exercises. They're ideal for home use.
- **Cardio Machines:** If you have the space, investing in a treadmill or stationary bike can be beneficial. Choose one based on your available space and cardio preferences.
- **Storage Solutions:** To keep your home gym organized, consider wall-mounted racks for resistance bands, dumbbells, or kettlebells and a designated area for a yoga mat.
- **Affordability:** With the right equipment, home workouts can be just as effective as gym workouts. Since you don't have to pay a membership fee, you can invest in quality gear over time.

b. Gym Setting Recommendations:

If you prefer working out at a gym, the key advantage is access to specialized equipment and professional guidance.

- **Variety of Equipment:** A gym provides access to various machines and free weights, such as leg presses, cable machines, and Olympic barbells, allowing you to train different muscle groups effectively.
- **Trainers and Classes:** Many gyms offer personal and group training, which can help beginners with form, progression, and motivation.

- **Gym Etiquette:** For those new to the gym environment, it's essential to familiarize yourself with gym etiquette, including wiping down equipment after use, sharing machines during busy times, and respecting others' workout space.

c. Cost Comparison (Home Gym vs. Gym Membership):

- **Initial Costs:** A home gym requires a higher initial investment, mainly if you buy a range of equipment. However, once purchased, you don't have recurring monthly fees.

- **Gym Membership Costs:** While a gym membership can be more affordable in the short term, it involves ongoing costs. Memberships may also be subject to initiation fees, cancellation fees, or annual increases.

- **Convenience:** Working out at home can be more convenient since you can exercise whenever you like. However, a gym might offer more variety and structured support, especially for beginners learning proper form and technique.

Conclusion

Fitness equipment is a critical factor in determining the success of your workout routine. Choosing the right gear at home or in the gym is essential for meeting your fitness goals and maintaining consistency. Beginners should start with the basics—like resistance bands, dumbbells, and a yoga mat—and progressively build their home gym or utilize gym facilities. When making decisions, consider your fitness goals, available space, and budget. You can ensure your fitness journey is enjoyable and effective with the right equipment.

Chapter 15: Incorporating Fitness into Busy Lifestyles

Introduction

Finding time to prioritize fitness can feel overwhelming in today's fast-paced world, where personal, professional, and social commitments are never-ending. However, maintaining an active lifestyle is crucial for physical health, mental well-being, and long-term vitality. This chapter addresses practical solutions for integrating fitness into a busy schedule, focusing on time management strategies, flexibility in routines, and creative ways to stay active during the day.

1. **Solutions for Time Management and Incorporating Short Workouts**

Effective time management is the cornerstone of making fitness part of a busy lifestyle. The key to fitting in workouts, even on the busiest days, lies in strategic planning, prioritizing, and smartly integrating fitness activities into everyday routines.

1. **Prioritize Fitness**

The first step to incorporating fitness into a busy lifestyle is recognizing its importance. Many people wait until their schedules open up, which often doesn't happen. Instead, fitness should be viewed as a non-negotiable priority, like eating, sleeping, or working. To make fitness a habit:

- **Set clear fitness goals**: Define short-term and long-term objectives, whether losing weight, building muscle, or improving cardiovascular health.
- **Schedule workouts as appointments**: Treat your workouts as important meetings that can't be rescheduled. Block out specific times in your calendar for exercise, and protect them like any other work meeting.

1. **Short Workouts**

When time is limited, it's essential to maximize the efficiency of workouts. While traditional gym sessions may take an hour or more, shorter, high-intensity workouts can offer significant benefits in less time.

- **High-Intensity Interval Training (HIIT)**: HIIT involves short bursts of intense exercise followed by short recovery periods. These workouts can be completed in as little as 20–30 minutes, and they improve cardiovascular health, strength, and endurance.
- **Circuit Training**: Circuit training involves performing exercises targeting different muscle groups with minimal rest between sets. This keeps the heart rate elevated and can be a highly efficient workout in a short period.
- **Tabata Training** is a specific form of HIIT that consists of 20 seconds of ultra-intense exercise and 10 seconds of rest for four minutes per exercise. It's a great way to burn fat and build strength quickly.

- **Bodyweight Workouts**: When pressed for time, bodyweight exercises can be done anywhere without equipment. Squats, push-ups, lunges, and planks are excellent exercises for short, effective workouts.

1. **Combine Workouts with Other Tasks**

Sometimes, it's about being clever with time. Here are a few ways to combine exercise with your other daily activities:

- **Walking or biking to work**: Instead of driving or taking public transport, walk or cycle to your destination. This incorporates low-intensity cardio into your daily routine.
- **Desk exercises**: If you're tied to a desk most of the day, incorporate stretches or seated exercises. Try chair squats, seated leg lifts, or stretching during phone calls or meetings.
- **Workouts during TV time**: Rather than just sitting on the couch, use commercial breaks or Netflix episodes as an opportunity to do a quick workout, such as push-ups, jumping jacks, or planks.

1. **Importance of Flexibility and Adaptability in Routine**

One of the main reasons many people struggle with maintaining a fitness routine is that life often gets in the way. Work may run late, kids may need attention, or other commitments might crop up unexpectedly. A rigid routine can cause frustration and lead to abandoning fitness goals. Flexibility and adaptability are crucial to making fitness a sustainable part of a busy lifestyle.

1. **Be Open to Adjusting Your Schedule**

When life gets unpredictable, having flexibility in your workout schedule is essential. If you can't make your morning workout, consider fitting it in during lunch or evening hours. Rather than stressing over missing a session, adapt and reschedule it.

- **Adjust based on energy levels**: If you're feeling exhausted one day, opt for a low-impact activity such as walking or yoga instead of pushing yourself through a high-intensity workout.
- **Prioritize consistency over perfection**: Even if you can only fit in 10 minutes of exercise today, it's better than doing nothing. Over time, consistency is vital to seeing results.

1. **Cross-Training and Variety**

Cross-training is another way to maintain flexibility in your fitness routine. By varying the exercise types, you keep your routine exciting and reduce the risk of burnout. It also helps prevent injury by not overusing the same muscle groups.

- **Mix-up workouts**: Alternate between strength training, cardio, flexibility exercises, and rest days. Try different activities like swimming, biking, yoga, or dancing to keep things fresh.
- **Adapt to seasonal changes**: In the winter, you may need to swap outdoor runs for indoor exercises, like using a treadmill or doing a home workout. In summer, outdoor activities like hiking, running, or playing sports can be great options.

1. **Build a Flexible Fitness Plan**

Your fitness plan should adapt to your life, not vice versa. A good approach is to:

- **Have a range of workout options**: Include options for different time constraints, such as a 20-minute HIIT workout, a 30-minute yoga flow, or a 45-minute weightlifting session.
- **Have backup plans**: Keep a set of at-home exercises or gym routines that don't require much equipment to work out at home.

1. **Creative Ways to Stay Active in Daily Life**

Staying active can sometimes mean going to the gym or setting aside 30 minutes for a workout. There are many creative and enjoyable ways to stay active throughout the day, turning everyday tasks into opportunities for fitness.

1. **Active Commuting**

For many people, commuting is a large portion of their day. Why not make the most of it by incorporating fitness into your commute?

- **Walking or cycling**: If your workplace is within walking or cycling distance, use that time for cardio.
- **Take the stairs**: Whenever possible, take the stairs instead of using the elevator. Climbing stairs is an excellent way to engage your legs and glutes.

1. **Fitness Breaks at Work**

Long hours at a desk can lead to stiffness and poor posture. Taking breaks for movement can help combat this.

- **Stretching**: Take 5–10 minutes to stand up and stretch your muscles every hour or so. Focus on the neck, shoulders, back, and legs to alleviate tension from sitting.
- **Walk and talk**: If you have a meeting or phone call, consider walking around the office or outside while talking. This can improve circulation and add to your daily steps.
- **Standing desks**: Consider using a standing desk or a convertible desk to alternate between sitting and standing during your workday.

1. **Household Chores as Exercise**

Household chores, often seen as mundane tasks, can provide a decent workout if done with intention.

- **Vacuuming and sweeping**: These activities can provide an aerobic workout while working your arms and legs.
- **Gardening**: Digging, planting, and weeding engage multiple muscle groups and can be a surprisingly effective way to stay active.

- **Washing dishes or folding laundry** might seem passive, but you can turn them into mini-workouts by focusing on posture, engaging your core, and adding dynamic movement.

1. **Social Activities**

Staying active doesn't have to be a solo endeavor. Many social activities can be physically engaging; involving friends or family can make fitness more enjoyable.

- **Playing sports**: Join a recreational league, play tennis, go bowling, or enjoy other sports with friends or family.
- **Active family outings**: Instead of meeting friends or family for a coffee or dinner suggest an activity like a hike, a walk in the park, or a bike ride.
- **Dance parties**: Whether at a party or at home, dancing is a fun and effective way to increase your heart rate.

1. **Small Lifestyle Changes**

Incorporating fitness into your daily routine can sometimes require drastic changes. Minor adjustments can make a big difference.

- **Stand while working**: Switch to a standing desk or use a high countertop for a few hours daily.
- **Use a pedometer or fitness tracker**: Tracking your steps can motivate you to move more. Aim for a daily step count, and find opportunities to walk more.

Conclusion

Incorporating fitness into a busy lifestyle requires careful planning, flexibility, and creativity. By managing time effectively, remaining adaptable in your routine, and finding innovative ways to stay active throughout the day, it's possible to maintain a healthy, active lifestyle without feeling overwhelmed. Remember, fitness is a journey, not a destination; every small effort contributes to long-term well-being. Whether you have 10 minutes or an hour, finding ways to prioritize movement can have lasting benefits for your physical and mental health.

Chapter 16: Exploring Advanced Training Techniques

1. **Introduction to Advanced Fitness Concepts:**

Advanced fitness techniques go beyond the foundational exercises that form the core of most training programs. These methods are designed to push physical limits, enhance performance, and engage muscles in novel ways. Two of the most prominent advanced techniques include **High-Intensity Interval Training (HIIT)** and **CrossFit**. Both methods have gained popularity due to their effectiveness and ability to achieve rapid results.

High-Intensity Interval Training (HIIT):

HIIT is a time-efficient training method that alternates between short bursts of intense activity and brief periods of low-intensity recovery or rest. It has become increasingly popular for its ability to improve cardiovascular health, build strength, and burn fat relatively quickly.

Key Features of HIIT:

- **Intensity:** You push yourself to your maximum effort during the work phase.
- **Intervals:** Work intervals are usually between 20-45 seconds, with rest periods ranging from 10-30 seconds.
- **Variety:** Exercises can range from bodyweight movements (like squat push-ups) to using equipment (such as kettlebells, resistance bands, or rowing machines).
- **Efficiency:** HIIT workouts can be completed in 20-30 minutes, making them ideal for individuals with busy schedules.

Benefits of HIIT:

- **Fat Loss:** HIIT is known for its ability to increase fat burn due to its high intensity, which leads to a higher post-exercise calorie burn (EPOC—Excess Post-exercise Oxygen Consumption).
- **Improved Cardiovascular Fitness:** Studies show that HIIT can improve VO2 max, a key indicator of cardiovascular fitness.
- **Metabolic Boost:** By increasing metabolic rate, HIIT helps sustain calorie burn even after the workout.

CrossFit:

CrossFit is a branded fitness regimen that incorporates exercises from different disciplines, such as Olympic weightlifting, gymnastics, and cardio. The program is designed to build strength, power, endurance, agility, and flexibility through constantly varied workouts.

Key Features of CrossFit:

- **Functional Movements:** The emphasis is on movements that mirror everyday tasks, such as lifting, jumping, running, and carrying.
- **Constant Variation:** Every workout is different, so participants never get bored or hit a plateau.
- **Scalability:** CrossFit is adaptable to all fitness levels. Movements and weights are scaled to match the individual's abilities, making it accessible even to beginners willing to progress at their own pace.

- **Community Focus:** CrossFit thrives on camaraderie. Group workouts and supportive coaching create a motivating environment.

Benefits of CrossFit:

- **Strength and Conditioning:** CrossFit combines aerobic exercise with strength training, improving overall fitness and functional strength.
- **Increased Performance:** CrossFit athletes typically excel in multiple fitness domains, including endurance, strength, and flexibility.
- **Motivation and Accountability:** CrossFit gyms' sense of community and competitive atmosphere help participants stay motivated and committed to their training goals.

1. **Benefits of Advanced Techniques and Potential Risks**

Advanced training techniques like HIIT and CrossFit offer substantial benefits but have potential risks that must be considered. Understanding these is crucial for safe training progression.

Benefits of Advanced Techniques:

- **Enhanced Cardiovascular Health:** HIIT and CrossFit push the cardiovascular system to its limits, improving heart and lung capacity. Over time, the heart becomes more efficient at pumping blood, which helps reduce the risk of heart disease and improve overall endurance.
- **Increased Strength and Muscle Mass:** These techniques, particularly CrossFit, focus on compound exercises like squats, deadlifts, and press variations that target multiple muscle groups, leading to significant increases in both strength and lean muscle mass.
- **Improved Functional Fitness:** Because CrossFit incorporates movements that simulate daily activities, athletes develop greater overall body awareness and functional strength, which enhances performance in everyday life.
- **Time Efficiency:** HIIT is especially popular because it delivers a high-calorie burn and increases metabolic rate quickly, making it ideal for people with time constraints.
- **Enhanced Metabolism:** HIIT and CrossFit can help increase metabolic rate for hours after the workout, burning more calories throughout the day (afterburn effect).
- **Mental Toughness:** The intensity of these workouts can help develop mental resilience. Pushing through fatigue and discomfort builds both physical and psychological endurance.

Potential Risks of Advanced Techniques:

- **Overtraining:** Advanced techniques place a lot of strain on the body. Without proper rest and recovery, individuals can experience overtraining syndrome, leading to fatigue, decreased performance, and even injury.
- **Injury Risk:** CrossFit's high-intensity and complex movements mainly increase the risk of injury if exercises are not performed correctly. Overuse injuries, such as tendinitis and stress fractures, can also occur from excessive repetition.

- **Cardiovascular Stress:** While beneficial for cardiovascular health, HIIT workouts can be risky for individuals with existing heart conditions. The high intensity of the exercises, coupled with minimal rest, can cause spikes in blood pressure and heart rate, which might not be safe for those with cardiovascular issues.
- **Muscle Imbalance:** The training intensity can lead to muscle imbalances if not balanced with appropriate recovery and complementary exercises. Overloading one muscle group without working with others can lead to poor posture and injury.
- **Mental Burnout:** The psychological strain of high-intensity workouts can lead to burnout or fatigue, particularly for those new to advanced techniques or those without adequate recovery.

1. **Guidance on Progressing Safely to Advanced Levels**

While advanced training techniques like HIIT and CrossFit are highly effective, they are not recommended for everyone, especially those just starting or those with pre-existing health issues. It's important to gradually progress towards these techniques with a structured approach that prioritizes safety.

Progressing Safely:

1. **Build a Strong Foundation:** Before diving into high-intensity techniques, it's essential to have a solid foundation in basic strength training and aerobic fitness. This ensures that the body is prepared for the intensity of advanced techniques. For example, focusing on mastering bodyweight exercises like push-ups, squats, and lunges can help build strength and stability before progressing to weighted exercises.
2. **Start with a Beginner-Friendly Version:** If you're new to HIIT or CrossFit, start with a beginner version of these workouts. Many CrossFit gyms offer "on-ramp" programs or intro courses designed to introduce new participants to the movements at a manageable pace. Similarly, HIIT workouts can be modified by reducing the intensity or duration of the intervals to prevent burnout.
3. **Gradual Progression:** The key to avoiding injury while progressing to advanced levels is gradual progression. Slowly increase the intensity, volume, and complexity of your workouts. In HIIT, for example, you might start with 20-second intervals of high intensity and increase the duration or intensity over time as your fitness improves.
4. **Focus on Proper Form:** Advanced techniques often involve complex and compound movements. It's crucial to perform exercises with correct form to reduce the risk of injury. Consider working with a coach or personal trainer to ensure you're executing exercises properly, particularly in CrossFit where Olympic lifting techniques are common.
5. **Incorporate Rest and Recovery:** Adequate rest is essential when progressing to more intense forms of training. Make sure you're giving your body enough time to recover between sessions, and listen

to your body when it signals fatigue. Active recovery days, stretching, foam rolling, and adequate sleep are all vital components of any successful advanced training regimen.

6. **Cross-Training:** While focusing on one type of advanced technique is fine, it's important to include variety to reduce the risk of overuse injuries. Cross-training involves mixing different styles of exercise to keep workouts interesting and challenging while giving specific muscle groups time to recover. For example, combining HIIT workouts with yoga or swimming can offer balance and flexibility to your training.

7. **Nutrition and Hydration:** Advanced training techniques demand more from your body, which means your nutritional needs are greater. Ensure you're fueling your body properly with sufficient protein for muscle recovery, carbohydrates for energy, and fats for overall health. Hydration is equally important, particularly during high-intensity workouts that lead to significant fluid loss.

8. **Listen to Your Body:** Finally, one of the most crucial aspects of progressing safely is listening to your body. Pay attention to any signs of discomfort or pain during workouts. If something feels off, stop and rest. Pushing through pain can lead to serious injuries that could sideline your progress.

Conclusion:

In conclusion, advanced training techniques like HIIT and CrossFit offer numerous benefits, including improved cardiovascular health, increased strength, and enhanced overall fitness. However, they also come with risks that can be mitigated through careful progression, proper form, and adequate recovery. By building a solid foundation, starting with beginner-friendly versions of these workouts, and paying attention to your body's signals, you can safely incorporate these advanced techniques into your fitness journey and reap their full benefits.

Chapter 17: Understanding the Science of Fitness

1. **Basic Overview of Exercise Physiology**

Exercise physiology is the study of the body's responses to physical activity and how various systems adapt to increased physical demands. It focuses on understanding the biochemical and physiological changes during and after Exercise and how the body adjusts over time with consistent training. This field explores the relationship between Exercise, physical performance, and overall health.

Exercise physiology involves understanding how energy production occurs within the body, how muscles respond to load and strain, how the cardiovascular and respiratory systems work during physical exertion, and how recovery processes arise. The study of exercise physiology also explores the factors influencing fitness levels, such as nutrition, genetics, environment, and age.

The Physiology of Exercise: Key Concepts

- **Homeostasis and Adaptation:** Homeostasis refers to the body's ability to maintain a stable internal environment. Exercise challenges this balance, and over time, the body adapts to exercise stress to optimize efficiency.
- **Energy Metabolism:** Exercise relies on various energy systems to fuel muscles. Understanding these systems is central to the science of fitness.
- **Muscle Contraction:** Muscles contract in response to electrical impulses, which is fundamental for all forms of Exercise, whether aerobic or anaerobic.
- **Oxygen Transport:** The efficiency of the body's delivery of oxygen to working muscles plays a significant role in endurance and performance.

1. **How Exercise Affects Different Bodily Systems**

Several physiological systems support and sustain the activity when we engage in physical activity. Exercise stimulates a cascade of body reactions, ultimately affecting every system. Below are the leading systems impacted by Exercise:

2.1 Musculoskeletal System

The musculoskeletal system consists of muscles, bones, and connective tissues and is responsible for the body's movement. Exercise enhances muscular strength, endurance, flexibility, and coordination.

- **Muscle Fiber Recruitment:** During Exercise, motor units are activated in a sequence depending on the intensity of the Exercise. Low-intensity exercises recruit slow-twitch fibers (Type I), which are fatigue-resistant but less powerful. High-intensity exercises recruit fast-twitch fibers (Type II), which generate more force but fatigue quickly.

- **Muscle Hypertrophy:** Regular strength training causes muscle fibers to grow in size, a process called hypertrophy. This is primarily due to increased protein synthesis within muscle cells, leading to muscle repair and growth after resistance training.
- **Bone Density:** Weight-bearing exercises like running, weightlifting, or resistance training stimulate bone remodeling, leading to increased bone mineral density and a reduced risk of osteoporosis.

2.2 Cardiovascular System

The cardiovascular system, consisting of the heart and blood vessels, delivers oxygen and nutrients to muscles and removes metabolic waste products such as carbon dioxide.

- **Cardiac Output:** During Exercise, the heart pumps more blood to meet the body's increased oxygen demands. This is achieved by an increase in heart rate (HR) and stroke volume (SV).
- **Blood Flow Redistribution:** Exercise increases blood flow to the muscles, skin, and heart while reducing blood flow to less active organs such as the digestive system.
- **Vascular Adaptations:** Regular aerobic Exercise makes blood vessels elastic, improving and reducing bloreducingsure. Long-term cardiovascular training increases density, enhancing oxygen and nutrient delivery to muscles.

2.3 Respiratory System

The respiratory system ensures the body gets enough oxygen and removes carbon dioxide produced during Exercise.

- **Ventilation and Breathing Rate:** During Exercise, the respiratory system works harder to meet the body's oxygen demands. Depending on the intensity of the Exercise, both the rate and depth of breathing increase significantly.
- **Oxygen Uptake:** Taking in and utilizing oxygen efficiently is crucial for endurance performance. Oxygen uptake (VO_2 max) is a key indicator of aerobic fitness and represents the maximum amount of oxygen the body can use during intense Exercise.
- **Lung Capacity and Efficiency:** Regular Exercise improves lung function by increasing vital capacity (the air the lungs can hold) and improving the efficiency with which oxygen is transferred from the lungs to the bloodstream.

2.4 Nervous System

The nervous system, comprising the brain, spinal cord, and peripheral nerves, coordinates muscle movement and the body's overall response to Exercise.

- **Motor Control:** The brain sends electrical impulses to muscles to initiate movement. Exercise improves neuromuscular efficiency, resulting in better coordination and motor control.
- **Central Nervous System (CNS) Fatigue:** Prolonged or high-intensity Exercise can lead to CNS fatigue, which reduces motor unit recruitment and overall performance. Overtraining can lead to chronic fatigue and affect performance.

2.5 Endocrine System

The endocrine system includes glands that produce hormones that regulate metabolism, growth, and recovery. Exercise significantly affects hormone levels, influencing energy balance and the body's ability to adapt to physical stress.

- **Insulin Sensitivity:** Regular physical activity improves insulin sensitivity, which helps regulate blood sugar levels and reduce the risk of type 2 diabetes.
- **Growth Hormone (GH) and Testosterone:** Growth hormone and testosterone levels rise during strength training. These hormones play vital roles in muscle repair, growth, and fat loss.
- **Cortisol and Stress Response:** Exercise increases cortisol, a hormone that helps the body manage stress. However, chronic high levels of cortisol due to overtraining can have adverse effects, including muscle breakdown and immune suppression.

1. **The Role of Hormones and Energy Systems in Fitness**

The body relies on different energy systems to produce the ATP (adenosine triphosphate) necessary for muscle contraction during Exercise. These energy systems are regulated by hormonal responses, which help ensure the body has enough fuel to sustain activity.

3.1 Energy Systems in Fitness

The body uses three primary energy systems to produce ATP during physical activity: the phosphagen system (ATP-PC), anaerobic glycolysis, and aerobic metabolism.

- **Phosphagen System (ATP-PC):** This system provides immediate energy for short bursts of intense activity, such as sprints or heavy lifts. It uses stored ATP and phosphocreatine (PCr) in the muscles to regenerate ATP rapidly. This system is dominant for activities lasting 10-15 seconds.
- **Anaerobic Glycolysis (Lactic Acid System):** This system kicks in for activities lasting between 30 seconds and 2 minutes. It breaks down glucose into pyruvate, producing ATP without requiring oxygen. However, this process also produces lactic acid, leading to muscle fatigue and discomfort.
- **Aerobic Metabolism:** The body primarily uses aerobic metabolism for prolonged activities, such as long-distance running or cycling. This system breaks down carbohydrates, fats, and sometimes proteins in the presence of oxygen to produce a large amount of ATP. It is the most efficient energy system and supports activities lasting over several minutes.

3.2 Hormonal Regulation of Energy Systems

Hormones play a crucial role in regulating energy systems during Exercise. Several essential hormones are involved:

- **Insulin:** Released from the pancreas, insulin helps regulate glucose and fat metabolism. During Exercise, insulin sensitivity increases, allowing for better glucose uptake into muscle cells for energy.
- **Glucagon:** Also produced by the pancreas, glucagon works in opposition to insulin. It helps release stored glucose from the liver

during Exercise, ensuring muscles have enough fuel for sustained activity.

- **Adrenaline (Epinephrine):** Released from the adrenal glands, adrenaline prepares the body for physical exertion by increasing heart rate, blood flow to muscles, and the breakdown of glycogen into glucose for quick energy.
- **Cortisol:** As mentioned earlier, cortisol helps mobilize energy stores during stress and Exercise. It increases glucose availability by promoting the breakdown of protein and fat, but high cortisol levels over time can be detrimental.
- **Testosterone and Growth Hormone:** These hormones are essential for muscle repair, hypertrophy, and recovery. They stimulate the synthesis of proteins and the growth of muscle fibers.

3.3 The Impact of Hormones on Performance and Recovery

The balance between anabolic (muscle-building) and catabolic (muscle-breaking) hormones is essential for fitness gains. While exercise-induced increases in cortisol are necessary for energy mobilization, excessive cortisol due to overtraining can hinder recovery and lead to muscle breakdown.

Testosterone, growth hormone, and insulin-like growth factor (IGF-1) promote muscle recovery and growth. Ensuring adequate recovery time between workouts allows for the optimal hormonal response that supports muscle adaptation and performance improvements.

3.4 Hormonal Fluctuations with Different Types of Exercise

- **Resistance Training:** Intense, short-duration activities like weight lifting cause an acute increase in testosterone and growth hormone levels, stimulating muscle growth and strength.
- **Endurance Exercise:** Longer, moderate-intensity Exercise, such as running or cycling, results in elevated cortisol levels, but with regular training, the body adapts to become more efficient at utilizing fat as fuel, reducing the reliance on glycogen and glucose.

Chapter 18: Community and Support in Fitness

1. Exploring the Benefits of Group Workouts and Fitness Communities Fitness is often perceived as an individual journey, where personal motivation, discipline, and self-direction are critical components to achieving goals. However, the importance of a community in the fitness world has become increasingly evident. Group workouts and fitness communities offer unique benefits that can enhance one's fitness experience, leading to tremendous long-term success and satisfaction. Let's explore these benefits in detail.

a) Motivation and Encouragement: One of the most significant advantages of group workouts and fitness communities is the motivation that stems from being surrounded by like-minded individuals. Humans are social creatures, and the presence of others can push us to achieve more than we would on our own. This is especially important when motivation wanes and staying consistent with personal fitness goals becomes harder.

Participants often push each other to complete a challenging exercise or surpass their limits in a group setting. The energy created in a group workout environment can foster a sense of camaraderie that encourages individuals to continue despite feeling tired or unmotivated.

b) Accountability: When we work out in a group, there's a certain level of accountability that isn't present when we work out alone. Having a workout buddy or being part of a fitness group creates an external sense of responsibility. Knowing that others depend on you to show up or that your attendance is being noticed can motivate individuals to stay consistent. This shared accountability enhances personal responsibility and strengthens relationships within the group.

c) Social Connections: Fitness communities offer an excellent opportunity to develop social bonds. Group workouts and fitness classes foster a sense of belonging, where individuals feel part of something larger than themselves. These connections can lead to lasting friendships, and having a social network with similar health and fitness values can encourage people to stay engaged with their fitness journey.

Furthermore, fitness communities often become supportive environments that extend beyond physical exercise, offering emotional support and even opportunities for professional networking.

d) Sense of Belonging and Support: Whether online or offline, fitness communities often focus on inclusivity and support. In these communities, members feel they belong to a group that understands their challenges and struggles. These groups provide a safe, non-judgmental environment where individuals can be themselves, share personal stories, and support one another through tough times.

e) Structured Programs and Guidance: Group fitness programs often include structured routines led by experienced instructors. These programs are designed to challenge participants while ensuring they follow a well-balanced approach to training. Having access to professional guidance within a group setting can help individuals achieve better results than relying solely on their own knowledge or intuition.

f) Fun and Enjoyment: Group workouts are more fun and dynamic than solitary workouts. Whether it's a dance class, a cycling group, or a CrossFit session, a unique energy makes exercise enjoyable. Having a good time while working out can enhance overall adherence to a fitness routine, especially for people who struggle with motivation to exercise on their own.

g) Competition and Friendly Rivalry: Healthy competition can motivate greatly. In group settings, friendly rivalry often encourages participants to perform better. This element of competition is typically rooted in respect and mutual encouragement, and it can drive participants to push harder, achieve their best, and feel a sense of accomplishment when they meet or exceed their goals.

1. Building a Personal Support System for Accountability

Creating a personal support system is essential for long-term fitness success. A strong network of people who encourage, guide, and hold you accountable can make the difference between success and failure. Here are several strategies for building an effective personal support system in your fitness journey.

a) Identifying Key Support Individuals: Your support system should consist of individuals who are committed to your success and who will encourage you to stay on track. This could be a family member, a close friend, a workout partner, or a fitness coach. The key is choosing people who understand your goals and will genuinely hold you accountable, not just give you excuses when you miss a workout.

A workout partner is particularly effective; you can attend sessions together, share the challenges, and provide mutual motivation. This social support system creates a bond that makes skipping workouts or falling off track harder.

b) Accountability Partnerships: One of the most effective ways to ensure consistency in your fitness routine is through accountability partnerships. This can be as simple as scheduling workouts with friends or partners. The concept is to commit to show up and exercise together. Knowing someone relying on you to attend can be a potent motivator.

Accountability partners can also check your progress, encourage you to meet milestones, and even help troubleshoot any issues. A good accountability partner understands your goals and offers constructive feedback, not just praise.

c) Setting Goals and Tracking Progress: Clarifying your goals is crucial to building a personal support system. These goals should be specific, measurable, and achievable. Sharing your fitness goals with your support system creates a sense of transparency and allows others to monitor your progress. Additionally, it will enable them to help you overcome obstacles and celebrate victories along the way.

Tracking progress is another essential element. Whether you're tracking your weight, body fat percentage, strength gains, or overall fitness level, regular check-ins with your support system can help you stay motivated and see the fruits of your hard work. Many fitness communities use apps or fitness trackers to log and share results with others.

d) Professional Support: While friends and family can be excellent sources of emotional support, professional guidance can make a significant difference in your fitness journey. Personal trainers, nutritionists, or physical therapists can provide expert advice tailored to your needs. A fitness professional can design a personalized training program, ensure that you're exercising with the proper form, and make adjustments to your routine as you progress.

Moreover, professional support also helps reduce the risk of injury and optimize your performance. Having a coach or trainer also adds an extra layer of accountability because you are committing to a scheduled session, and they will help guide you through the process.

e) Online Fitness Communities: The digital age has made building a personal support system more accessible. Online fitness communities provide a platform for individuals to connect, share progress, ask questions, and motivate each other. Social media groups, fitness apps, and forums allow instant access to information, resources, and moral support.

For instance, joining a Facebook group for a specific fitness goal (e.g., weight loss, strength training, marathon preparation) allows you to share challenges, seek advice, and celebrate wins with people worldwide. These online platforms create a sense of camaraderie and help you stay connected with others who share similar goals and struggles.

1. Accessing Online Resources and Communities

In today's world, online resources and communities are invaluable for anyone pursuing a fitness journey. They not only provide access to information and tools but also offer emotional support, motivation, and accountability from people all over the world. Let's delve deeper into how to access and use these resources effectively.

a) Fitness Apps: A wide range of fitness apps are available, each designed to meet different needs. Whether you're looking for strength training programs, cardio workouts, or yoga classes, there's an app for nearly every type of exercise. Some popular apps include:

- **MyFitnessPal** – Used for tracking diet and exercise.
- **Strava** – Ideal for runners and cyclists to track routes and connect with others.
- **Nike Training Club** – Offers free workouts designed by professional trainers.
- **Fitbit** – Tracks physical activity and provides motivation and health insights.

These apps often have social features, allowing users to connect with friends and other users, share progress, and challenge one another. Some apps even allow for live interaction with coaches or fitness experts.

b) social media and Fitness Influencers: Social media platforms like Instagram, YouTube, and TikTok have become hubs for fitness enthusiasts, influencers, and experts. You can get inspiration, workout ideas, and motivational content by following fitness influencers. Many fitness influencers share workout routines, nutrition tips, and personal fitness journeys, which can help you stay inspired.

In addition, social media platforms allow for direct engagement, enabling you to ask questions, comment on posts, and participate in live sessions or Q&As. The interactive nature of these platforms builds a sense of community where followers can connect and share their experiences.

c) Online Fitness Classes and Programs: Online fitness classes are an excellent resource for those who prefer to work out at home or cannot access a gym. Platforms like Peloton, Beachbody on Demand, and other streaming services offer live or on-demand classes. These platforms have options for beginners and advanced participants, and many provide group features where users can interact with instructors or fellow participants.

Moreover, many fitness websites and apps offer free or low-cost access to professional-led fitness programs, which can be followed at your own pace. This convenience makes it easier to stay consistent, as you can follow structured programs that fit your schedule and lifestyle.

d) Virtual Fitness Communities: Online communities like Reddit, Discord, or Facebook groups have become a valuable resource for those seeking support and advice in their fitness journey. These platforms allow users to post questions, share accomplishments, and seek advice from experts and peers.

Virtual fitness communities also provide a sense of belonging, where individuals can find accountability partners or workout buddies.

Chapter 19: Expert Insights and Success Stories

1. **Inspirational Stories from Individuals Who Transformed Their Lives Through Fitness**

This section highlights personal transformation stories—individuals who have overcome obstacles, pushed through adversity, and used fitness to change their lives drastically. These stories are meant to inspire and show readers that fitness isn't just about physical changes; it's a journey of self-discovery, empowerment, and sometimes even spiritual awakening.

a) The Power of Resilience – A Journey from Obesity to Marathon Runner

One of the most compelling stories might be about someone who was once morbidly obese, struggling with self-esteem and health issues like high blood pressure, diabetes, and sleep apnea. Overcoming these challenges requires more than just physical transformation; it takes mental strength, a supportive environment, and a clear goal. This person may have started walking on a treadmill, gradually increasing distance and intensity, eventually building up to running a full marathon. Through consistent training and adopting healthier eating habits, they could have reversed their diabetes, lost a significant amount of weight, and transformed their body and lives.

b) Overcoming Injury – From Paralysis to Strength Training

Another powerful transformation story might involve someone who faced a severe injury—such as a spinal cord injury—that left them with limited mobility or even paralysis. The road to recovery could have been extended and fraught with physical therapy. Still, with the help of fitness professionals, adaptive equipment, and a relentless mindset, this person may have gradually regained strength, mobility, and confidence. Their journey highlights the power of fitness in rehabilitation, showing that even those told they might never walk again can experience life-changing results through persistence and proper training.

c) Rebuilding after Addiction – Fitness as a Tool for Recovery

For someone recovering from substance abuse or addiction, fitness can serve as an integral part of the recovery process. Physical activity releases endorphins, which help to combat the depression and anxiety often associated with addiction recovery. One such story could involve an individual who was battling alcohol or drug addiction and turned to fitness as a way to regain control over their life. Through dedication to regular workouts, they regained their physical health and gained mental clarity and emotional stability, eventually becoming an advocate for fitness within the recovery community.

d) Weight Loss through Sustainable Lifestyle Changes

Another transformative journey could focus on sustainable weight loss through a balanced diet and exercise. This individual may have struggled with yo-yo dieting for years, only to realize that weight loss comes from a holistic approach—incorporating a consistent exercise routine, mindful eating habits, and a positive mindset. Their story shows that while weight loss can be challenging, the long-term solution lies in sustainable habits supporting physical and mental health.

1. **Insights and Tips from Fitness Professionals**

In this section, we explore expert advice from fitness professionals. These tips are intended to help readers achieve their fitness goals and adopt a healthy lifestyle that supports long-term well-being.

a) Setting Realistic Goals and Tracking Progress

One key piece of advice from fitness experts is the importance of setting realistic and measurable goals. Fitness professionals often emphasize that goals should be specific, measurable, achievable, relevant, and time-bound (SMART). For instance, instead of setting a vague goal like "lose weight," a more specific goal would be "lose 10 pounds in 3 months by exercising 4 times a week and eating a balanced diet." Tracking progress helps maintain motivation and allows for adjustments along the way.

Fitness professionals recommend journaling workouts, taking progress photos, or using fitness tracking apps to monitor results over time. Tracking isn't just about physical progress; it also includes tracking mental well-being and mood changes, which are often overlooked.

b) The Importance of Strength Training

Experts often highlight the importance of strength training, especially for individuals looking to lose weight or increase their metabolic rate. Strength training doesn't just build muscle—it also improves bone density, boosts metabolism, and enhances overall functionality. Compound movements like squats, deadlifts, and bench presses are recommended, as they engage multiple muscle groups and help create a balanced, muscular body.

Many fitness professionals suggest a program that includes strength training and cardiovascular exercise to optimize results. Alternating between weightlifting sessions and cardio sessions like running, cycling, or swimming provides comprehensive fitness that targets different areas of the body.

c) Mind-Muscle Connection

A tip that experienced trainers often share is the importance of the mind-muscle connection during exercise. Fitness professionals emphasize that focusing on the muscles being worked during an exercise can led to more efficient and effective workouts. For example, rather than simply going through the motions of a bicep curl, the idea is to focus on contracting the biceps throughout the movement, which results in better activation of the muscle fibers and, ultimately, better growth.

d) Nutrition's Role in Fitness

Fitness professionals often advise that fitness is 80% nutrition and 20% exercise. Proper nutrition is the fuel that powers a workout and supports recovery afterward. Fitness experts usually recommend a diet rich in lean proteins, healthy fats, complex carbohydrates, and plenty of water to stay hydrated. They also suggest that people should eat based on their workout schedules—eating a small meal or snack that includes protein and carbs about 30-60 minutes before exercising and refueling with a post-workout meal that includes protein and carbs to repair and replenish muscle.

e) Recovery and Rest Days

Rest and recovery are just as important as exercise, and fitness professionals stress the importance of taking rest days and practicing active recovery. Overtraining can lead to burnout, injuries, and even a decline in performance. Recovery practices include stretching, yoga, foam rolling, massage therapy, or light walking. Sleep is also a crucial part of recovery, with many experts recommending 7-9 hours of sleep per night to allow the body time to repair itself.

f) Consistency Over Perfection

Fitness experts stress that consistency is more important than perfection. The idea that you must work out perfectly every time or eat a clean diet is unrealistic. It's more about showing up regularly, even when you don't feel like it, and sticking to the plan over time. By being consistent, individuals can see gradual improvements and long-lasting results.

1. **Learning from the Journeys of Others**

This section focuses on the valuable lessons that can be learned from the experiences of others who have successfully navigated fitness challenges.

a) The Role of Support Systems

One key takeaway from many successful fitness journeys is the importance of having a strong support system. Whether it's a workout buddy, a personal trainer, family members, or an online fitness community, support helps keep individuals accountable, motivated, and encouraged. Many success stories highlight the role of a fitness coach or group in pushing individuals to stay on track, particularly when they face moments of doubt or frustration.

b) The Mental and Emotional Benefits of Fitness

Many people find that fitness provides more than just physical benefits; it also supports emotional and mental well-being. Physical exercise has been shown to reduce anxiety, improve mood, and combat depression by releasing endorphins—the body's natural "feel-good" hormones. Learning from others' journeys, individuals can see how fitness is a tool for building self-confidence, managing stress, and improving mental health overall.

c) Overcoming Plateaus and Staying Motivated

Everyone reaches a point where progress slows down or even stalls entirely—a phenomenon known as a fitness plateau. Learning from others who have gone through this, individuals can see how they've overcome these plateaus. Whether changing their workout routine, adjusting their nutrition, or simply sticking with it despite setbacks, these stories offer encouragement and practical advice for anyone stuck.

d) Embracing the Process, Not Just the Results

A critical lesson from many success stories is the importance of focusing on the process rather than only the end goal. Fitness is not just about the destination (such as reaching a certain weight or body shape); it's about enjoying the journey and feeling more robust, energized, and confident along the way. Learning to embrace the small victories and personal growth that come with each workout can help individuals stay motivated in the long term.

Conclusion

Chapter 19, "Expert Insights and Success Stories," inspires and guides readers by showcasing real-life transformations and offering professional advice on how to approach fitness. By learning from others' journeys and heeding expert tips, individuals can better understand the importance of consistency, proper nutrition, strength training, and mental well-being in achieving their fitness goals. Fitness is a lifelong journey, and these stories and insights remind readers that transformation is not just physical—it is deeply rooted in perseverance, mindset, and support.

Feel free to ask if you need more details on any of the sections or additional content!

Chapter 20: Your Fitness Journey Begins Now

Introduction: Starting or Continuing the Fitness Journey

The title "Your Fitness Journey Begins Now" is a powerful and immediate call to action. This chapter is likely the culmination of everything the reader has learned in the previous chapters. It serves as the book's motivational conclusion, urging readers to take the first step (or perhaps the next) in their fitness journey, no matter where they are starting. The message is clear: there is no better time to begin than now, and the best time to act is always the present.

Starting a fitness journey can be daunting for many. The chapter acknowledges this fear and uncertainty and addresses people's common obstacles when considering a lifestyle change. These might include:

- **Fear of failure**: People often worry they will start a new fitness plan and not stick with it. They might fear they won't see results slowly, which leads to discouragement and giving up.
- **Lack of time**: Many people use lack of time as an excuse to delay their fitness journey. This chapter reassures readers that even small efforts can yield significant long-term results.
- **Feeling overwhelmed**: The vast amount of information available on fitness can be paralyzing. This chapter simplifies things, encouraging readers to take it one step at a time and focus on the basics first.
- **Physical limitations**: Many people feel that they are "too old," "too out of shape," or "too busy" to start a fitness routine. The chapter reminds readers that fitness is about progression, not perfection. Everyone can start at their own pace.

The chapter encourages readers to understand that starting a fitness journey does not require extreme changes or perfection. It's about progress, not perfection; any small change toward a healthier lifestyle is a win. Readers are encouraged to identify their reasons for wanting to get fit—whether it's to feel more energized, improve health, gain confidence, or be a role model for others—and remember these reasons when facing setbacks.

Summary of Key Takeaways from the Book

By the time the reader reaches Chapter 20, they have likely absorbed a wealth of information regarding fitness, nutrition, mindset, and the importance of consistency. Here's a breakdown of the key takeaways that might be summarized in this chapter:

1. **Fitness is a Lifelong Commitment**
2. Fitness is not a temporary fix or a "quick fad"; it's a lifelong journey. Building strength, endurance, and a healthy lifestyle requires commitment over time. Readers are encouraged to approach fitness as an ongoing, long-term habit rather than a short-term goal.
3. **Consistency is Key**
4. A primary emphasis throughout the book is the importance of consistency. Fitness progress is not achieved through bursts of

intense effort but through regular, sustainable actions over time. Whether exercising three times a week or making healthier food choices every day, the consistency in these small efforts will add up.

5. **Start Where You Are**
6. Another important theme is that fitness doesn't require starting at an elite level. Everyone's fitness journey is unique, and starting slow is okay. Whether you're a beginner or returning to fitness after a long hiatus, the goal is to take that first step. Gradual progress and setting realistic goals will help avoid discouragement.
7. **Physical Activity is Not Just About Appearance**
8. Many people approach fitness with the primary goal of changing their appearance. While body transformation can be a positive side effect of exercise, the main focus should be improving overall health—enhancing cardiovascular fitness, strength, flexibility, and mental clarity. Fitness should be seen as a way to improve overall well-being, not just aesthetics.
9. **The Importance of Recovery**
10. Recovery is just as important as the workouts themselves. The book likely emphasizes the importance of giving the body time to rest and rebuild. Sleep, stretching, and active recovery are all crucial components of a successful fitness journey. Overtraining can lead to burnout and injury, so balancing hard work with adequate rest is essential.
11. **Mindset Drives Results**
12. Mental attitude is one of the critical determinants of fitness success. The book stresses that adopting a positive mindset can help overcome obstacles. Mindset affects how one approaches workouts and how one handles setbacks or challenges along the way. A growth mindset, where challenges are viewed as opportunities to learn and improve, is critical to success.
13. **Nutrition Fuels Fitness**
14. Fitness and nutrition go hand in hand. The importance of fueling the body with the proper nutrients to support physical activity cannot be overstated. This includes a balanced diet rich in whole foods, lean proteins, healthy fats, and complex carbohydrates. Hydration also plays a critical role in optimizing workout performance and recovery.
15. **Set Achievable Goals**
16. Goal setting is used throughout the book to help readers track progress and stay motivated. Goals should be SMART (Specific, Measurable, Achievable, Relevant, and Time-bound). They give readers a clear direction, something to work towards, and a sense of achievement when milestones are met.
17. **Celebrate Every Victory**
18. The journey is just as important as the destination. Readers are reminded to celebrate small victories, whether increasing the weight lifted, running a longer distance, or simply sticking to the routine for a few weeks. These small wins are what ultimately lead to long-term success.

19. **Find Support and Accountability**
20. Fitness is often more enjoyable and sustainable when you have a support system. This could be through workout buddies, online communities, or fitness professionals like personal trainers. Accountability helps keep people on track and motivated, especially when things get tough.

Final Motivational Message to Inspire Readers

The closing part of Chapter 20 is designed to be an inspiring, uplifting message that spurs readers into action. Readers should feel equipped and motivated to continue or begin their journey after reading about the principles of fitness and the importance of consistency. Here's an example of a possible motivational message that could be included:

"Your Fitness Journey Begins Now"

No matter where you are in your fitness journey, remember that it's always possible to start, and you've already taken the first step by picking up this book. The path ahead may not always be easy, but it is always worth it. Every workout, every meal, and every small change you make adds up. Fitness is not about being perfect; it's about progress. It's about doing your best with what you have and where you are.

You are capable of more than you think. Your body is more vital than you realize, and your mind has the power to overcome any obstacle that stands in your way. Remember, fitness is not a destination—it's a journey. And the best part? You are already on the road.

Keep going, keep striving, and never forget why you started. You've got this."

Conclusion

Chapter 20 serves as both a culmination and a call to action for readers to put everything they've learned into practice. The key message is that fitness is a journey that requires persistence, patience, and a mindset focused on progress rather than perfection. It encourages readers to embrace where they are right now, to take the next step, and to keep moving forward. Whether starting from scratch or looking to continue their journey, the book leaves readers with the understanding that they can achieve their fitness goals one step at a time.

Let me know if you want further elaboration on any of these points or a more in-depth version!

Conclusion

Congratulations on completing The Ultimate Fitness Handbook: Transform Your Life! You've taken the first critical steps towards unlocking your full potential, and now it's time to put the knowledge you've gained into action. Throughout this book, we've covered the essential elements of fitness: exercise, nutrition, mindset, and recovery. These components are all crucial to creating a balanced, sustainable fitness plan. But remember, knowledge alone doesn't create transformation. Your commitment and consistency will lead to real, lasting change. As you move forward with your fitness journey, keep these key takeaways in mind:

- **Consistency is Key:** Fitness is not a short-term goal; it's a lifelong journey. Progress may seem slow at times, but persistence will always pay off.

- **Mindset Drives Results:** Your attitude towards fitness and life can make or break your success. Cultivate a positive mindset, stay motivated, and embrace growth challenges.

- **Nutrition Fuels Performance:** Your body needs the right fuel to perform. Focus on whole, nutrient-dense foods to power your workouts and support recovery.

- **Recovery Is Essential:** Don't underestimate the importance of rest. Allow your body time to recover, rebuild, and come back stronger.

The Ultimate Fitness Handbook is more than just a guide. It's a blueprint for lasting change. Now, it's up to you to take the next step. Whether you are beginning your fitness journey or looking to refine your existing routine, use the strategies you've learned to make healthier, more informed daily decisions. Thank you for trusting The Ultimate Fitness Handbook to be a part of your transformation. I'm confident that you will achieve the results you've always dreamed of with dedication and the right mindset. Keep moving forward, stay committed, and transform your life one step at a time. Your journey to a healthier, stronger, and more confident you start now.

Thank You